A Trainer's Guide for Preclinical Courses in Medicine

A Trainer's Guide for Preclinical Courses in Medicine

Tabitha Rangara-Omol

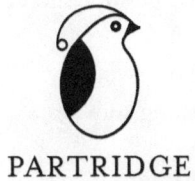

PARTRIDGE

ISBN: Softcover   978-1-4828-9993-1
                eBook   978-1-4828-9998-6

Print information available on the last page.

To order additional copies of this book, contact
Toll Free 800 101 2657 (Singapore)
Toll Free 1 800 81 7340 (Malaysia)
orders.singapore@partridgepublishing.com

www.partridgepublishing.com/singapore

Contents

Preface 1

Domains of Competencies 2

Acronyms 3

Introduction to the Trainer's Guide... 5

Templates and Samples within the Trainer's Guide 6

Training Module Guide Template... 7

Presentation Notes Template 8

Lesson Plan Template... 9

Curriculum Competency Objective and Assessment Matrix....10

Preclinical Courses (Introductory Block)..................................16

Course Description 16

Course Design 16

Module / Block Objective 16

Section I
Biomedical Sciences

Section IA Biomedical Sciences Classroom Learning 18

Anatomy 19

Histology 22

Embryology 27

Physiology.. 30

Biochemistry..37

Pathology 40

Microbiology.. 46

Immunology 54

Pharmacology 58

Section IB Integrated Biomedical Laboratory Practice........................ 64

Integrated Laboratory Sessions in Preclinical Courses 65

Planning for Demonstrations 65

Gross Anatomy 66

Histology 67

Embryology 68

Physiology..69

Biochemistry..70

Pathology 71

Microbiology and Parasitology 72

Pharmacology 73

Section II

Professional Competency Development (PCD)

PCD Course Description and Course Design 76

Course overview...76

Design...76

Section IIA Professional Competency Development Courses.............. 77

Introduction to Learning Methods...78

Study Skills 80

History of Medicine in the World and the context country 84

Clinical Skills... 86

Ethics and Legal Medicine 90

Professionalism... 94

Communication Skills 96

Essentials of ICT Skills 99

Evidence Based Medicine...102

First Aid..105

Section IIB Professional Competency Development...........................107

Clinical Skills Lab and Hospital OPD Practice 107

Demonstrations..108

Example I Procedure/Task: Medical History Taking..............................108

Example II Procedure/Task: Measuring Blood Pressure (Manually) 113

Additional teaching and learning methods 115

Time Table for Professional Competency Development for CVS:
    Clinical Skills Lab and Hospital OPD Practice...............................116

Section III
Social Population Health and Health Systems

Course Description 120

Course Design 120

Section IIIA Social Population Health and Health Systems.................121

Determinants of Health 122

Teaching-Learning Methods 126

Assessments..127

Resources Needed 127

Preface

A competency based curriculum is imperative to all health sciences and medical courses. The aim of any medical curriculum should be to provide student with training opportunities in the development of skills requisite to medical practice. A trainer's guide should be included as one of the training packages and units of competencies provided for by medical curricula. A training package is a set of nationally endorsed qualifications, competency standards and assessment guidelines that describe the skills and knowledge needed for medical personnel to perform effectively. To support the implementation of the curriculum, trainer's guides are provided so that the teacher has a quick reference and ready assistance in implementing curriculum activities. This training guide, therefore, incorporates the following unique concepts:

- Competencies are intentionally recognized as the basis of the curriculum implementation, delivery and assessment
- Different sciences are integrated at varying details at all levels of training.
- Education is integrated with practice in laboratory, health care facility and the community at every level.
- It has a design that implements early clinical contact and longitudinal community based education,
- It introduces innovative learning and teaching methodologies which encourage critical inquiry, self-reflection and team building
- Formative and summative assessments are used to improve continuous learning of student.

- It incorporates intentional emphasis on emergency surgical and life-saving skills, infectious diseases, rural health problems and national health priorities.
- It recognizes inter and trans professional education.
- It can easily be adapted for web- based learning and e-resources for student and faculty.

Domains of Competencies

There are seven domains of competencies addressed throughout this trainer's guide:

1. Scientific foundation of medicine
2. Clinical skills
3. Critical thinking and research and practice-based improvement
4. Communication skills
5. Professional values, attitudes, behavior and ethics
6. Population health and health systems
7. Management of information

Acronyms

CDs	Compact discs
COBE	Community Based Education
COME	Community Orientation in Medical Education
CPD	Continuing Professional Development
CRL	Computer Resource Learning
DOCS	Direct Observation of Clinical Skills
DVDs	Digital Versatile Discs
GPs	General Practitioners
Hrs	Hours
IL	Integrated learning
IS	Independent study
L	Lectures
MoH	Ministry of Health
OSCE	Objective Structured Clinical Examination
OSPE	Objective Structured Practical Examination
PBL	Problem-based Learning
PCD	Professional Competency Development
PRRE	Personal Research and Reflection Exercise
SDL	Self-Directed Learning
SGS	Small group sessions
SPH	Social and Population Health
VCDs	Versatile Compact Discs
WGS	Whole group sessions
WHO	World Health Organization
Wks	Weeks

Introduction to the Trainer's Guide

This trainer's guide provides guidelines but not hard rules for conducting training for each module or individual session. As a trainer, you are free to add practical ideas if they are within the scope of the curriculum. The length of each section in this trainer's guide depends on the number of modules or topics in your syllabus. In general, all information except those of the presentation notes is written in point format within the module or topic. This will include:

- **Topic title**
- **Resources**: List of materials required. List of materials for the module or individual training session, (e.g., audio-visual materials, hand-outs, training exercises).
- **Duration**: Length of the module or individual session
- **Competency Objectives Matrix**:
  o Competency objective, teaching methods and assessment methods matrix has been developed...
  o An outline of the relationship of the lesson to the course and/or the practice of medicine.
- **Assessment**: The measurements of the accomplishment of expected outcomes. The methods of measurement aim at your validation that each trainee exits from the system with ALL requisite competencies.
- **Lectures**:
  o Should provide clear inter-relationships of concepts, are interactive and if possible ask the student to draw a mind map to improve his/her mental image.
  o Presentation notes should also be provided.

- **Scheduling**: A chronological list of the sequence of activities or pieces of information / occurrences within the specific week of the module / course should be presented to the trainee(s).
- **Presentation notes**: The presentation notes can be written using a variety of styles. For example:
  o Columns, with cues in one column, (e.g., Hand-outs, training exercises, and visual-aid indicators that act as reminders and include various activities), and training content in the other column with indentation and bullets to identify key points.
  o Ensure that the notes are legible at a glance and designed to ensure you complete the key points of a particular module or topic.

Templates and Samples within the Trainer's Guide

Templates and samples are also provided in the trainer's guide. These templates are intended to provide support to the approach used to produce the training instruction materials. You may include notes or own comments / observations / reminders within your copy of the trainer's guide. The prescribed templates and samples included herein are:

1. Training module guide template
2. Presentation notes template
3. Lesson plan template

Training Module Guide Template

This template is used to document summary information applicable to a particular training module (see Table 1). The trainer's guide may already be filled in but there is no limit for you to add in practical ideas which may assist you in facilitating your student to gain the expected outcomes (competencies).

Table 1: Training Module Guide Sample

Program Title:			
Module Title:	**Module Code:**	**Module Duration:**	
Level of Study:			
Course / Subject:			
Duration of Course / Subject:			
Course Objectives		List clear specific and measurable objectives of what student are expected to achieve	
Measurement based on Module Objectives		List of assignments, tests, examinations and assessments.	
Relevance to Course / other modules / to practice		Outline as a reminder how this course builds to overall competencies	
Training Exercises		List of exercises which help the student in knowledge, skills and attitudes for this module/course.	
Materials Required		List of other required materials for this module	
Student Hand outs		List of student hand-outs for this module	
Audio-Visual Materials		List of audio-visual materials for the module	
Special Equipment		List of special equipment for this module	
Reference Materials		List all references materials where student can access further information	

Presentation Notes Template

You will use this template to document the sequence in which training information will be presented and to provide notes to remind yourself of the training content. In many ways, it resembles a lesson plan but has far less mandatory procedures. In any case, it is for optional use: an experienced trainer may not need it. This template may be used for each training module / course as sequenced in the trainer's guide.

Table 2: Presentation Notes Template Sample

Module/Course No/ Name / Code	
Sequence of presentation	**Presentation Notes**
1.1. Lesson Introduction	Provide a brief introduction to the lesson.
1.2. Purpose of Lesson	State purpose of the lesson.
1.3. Objective of Lesson	State objective of the lesson. • Indicate importance of the course / lesson. • Ask student for their ideas regarding the course / lesson.
1.4. Content of Lesson	Present details / discussions.
1.5. Lesson Exercise	Describe lesson exercise / demonstration / activities etc.
1.6. Review the Lesson / End	• Describe the relationship of the lesson to the previous lesson and the next lesson. • Provide exercises for review and reflection. • Assignments (optional)
1.7. Give an advance organizer	• Give a briefing of the next lesson.

Lesson Plan Template

A lesson plan is your detailed description of the course of instruction for **one individual lesson**. You are required to develop a daily lesson plan, as need be, to guide you during class instruction. Details will vary depending on your preferences, subject to be taught and the need and/or curiosity of the student. There may be requirements mandated by the curriculum but ultimately you have the freedom and style to choose the most effective methodology in delivering the learning materials to the student (see Table 3).

Table 3: Lesson Plan Template Sample

Module Name / No:		Topic / Subject:			
Duration:		Date:			
Course Level:	Course/ Subject:	Trainer's Name:			
Learning Outcomes: o o		Related Competencies: Refer the curriculum o o			
	Trainer's Guide	Student's Guide	Time limit	Resources	
Objectives Specify what the student will attain by the end of the lesson				Materials specific to the lesson e.g. Stationeries, multimedia equipment, LCD etc.	
Information / Content Give and/or demonstrate the necessary information.					
Verification Make steps to check for student understanding				Other resources e.g. Web, manikins, models	
Activity Make an independent activity to reinforce the lesson.					
Summary Recap the content and review the materials with the student				Additional resources and references	

Curriculum Competency Objective and Assessment Matrix

This is a guide detailing the seven domains of competencies which should be integrated all teaching and learning activities. There are seven domains of competencies addressed in the matrix (see Table 4):

1. Scientific foundation of medicine
2. Clinical skills
3. Critical thinking and research and practice-based improvement
4. Communication skills
5. Professional values, attitudes, behavior and ethics
6. Population health and health systems
7. Management of information

Table 4: Curriculum Competency Objective and Assessment Matrix

Competencies for Medical Doctors	Introduction to Medicine Competency / Objectives	Modules /activity /attachments	Teaching learning methods	Assessment
1. Scientific foundation of medicine	Student will be able to: • Identify the normal structure (Gross & Microscopic) and function of the body. • Describe molecular, cellular, biochemical and physiological mechanisms that maintain human body's Homeostasis and the intrinsic control mechanisms. • Explain the abnormalities in body structure and function of the human body which occur in diseased states and aging. • Distinguish gross and microscopic alterations of the body that occur in major pathologies and conditions. • Describe the major pathologic processes and the specific biological alterations which they cause. • Explain the aetiology and natural history of acute illnesses and chronic diseases. • Explain various causes of disorders and their pathogenesis. • Explain the normal and abnormal functions of human immunology.	Introduction to medicine modules. • Hospital visit • PHC unite visit	• Interactive Lecture • PBL • WGS • Integrated biomedical laboratory • E-learning • Mentorship • Self-Directed Learning • Community learning session	• Written exam • Viva • OSPE • 360°(Faculty observation and feedback)

	• Describe the human life cycle and effects of growth, development and aging upon the individual family and community. • Describe the principles of drug action and their use as well as the efficiency of various therapies. • Classify and describe commonly used drugs. • Use biomedical laboratories to understand the biomedical sciences.			• OSCE • 360°(Faculty observation and feedback) • Portfolios • OSPE • Global rating
2. Clinical skills	Student will be able to: • Explain the principles and practice taking an appropriate history in skill laboratory. • Explain the principles and practice to physical examination of the human body in skill laboratory and observe in hospital. • Observe and practice basic laboratory and biochemical tests. • Exercise basic laboratory experiment relevant to understanding biomedical science.	Introduction to medicine modules. • Hospital visit • PHC unit visit	• Interactive Lecture • SGS • WGS • Integrated biomedical lab • E-learning • Mentorship • Self-Directed Learning • Hospital and PHC visits	
3. Critical thinking and research Practice-based improvement,	Student will be able to: • Demonstrate a critical approach, constructive scepticism, creativity and a research-oriented attitude in professional activities;	Introduction to medicine modules. • Hospital visit • PHC unite visit	• SGS • PBL • WGS • E-learning • Self-Directed Learning	

	Learning Objectives	Content	Teaching/Learning Methods	Assessment
	• Recognize the power and limitations of the scientific thinking based on information obtained from different sources in establishing the causation, treatment and prevention of disease; • Experience practice-based improvement activities using a systematic methodology. • Use information technology to deepen one's own learning on the specific system. • Practice critically reviewing literature related to their learning. • Identify strategies to continuously update their knowledge and skills. • Systematically appraise and assimilate scientific evidence through reading of articles related to their learning. • Practice a habit of self-reflection, responsiveness to feedback and an on-going development of new skills, knowledge and attitude. • Excises self-motivation and accountability for own learning and facilitate the learning of other student and health care professionals.		• Hospital Visits • PHC weekly Visit • Community Learning Sessions	• Written exam • Portfolios • 360°(Faculty observation and feedback, peer evaluation) • PRRE
4. Communication skills	Student will be able to: • Use techniques which foster effective communication. • Apply basic communication skills to establish understanding with peers, faculty/staff, patient and their families.	Introduction to medicine modules. • Hospital visit • PHC unit visit	• Interactive Lectures • Role play • Role modelling • Mentorship • SGS	• Student presentation. • DOCS • 360°(Faculty feedback and observation, peer evaluation)

Theme	Learning outcomes	Content	Teaching/learning methods	Assessment methods
	• Interact with peers and other health professionals as an effective team member. • Listen attentively to elicit and compile relevant information from a patient. • Communicate effectively and demonstrate caring and respectful behaviours when interacting with patients and their families. • Write and orally present relevant information obtained from a patient. • Maintain good records. • Demonstrate sensitivity to cultural and personal factors that improve interactions with, patients, the community, peers and faculty. • Synthesize and present information appropriate to the needs of their learning, audience, and discuss plans of action.		• WGS • Hospital and PHC weekly visits • Skills laboratory	• Student presentation • Portfolios • Global Rating • 360° (Faculty observation and feedback, Peer evaluation)
5. Professionalism, ethics, behaviour and attitudes	Student will be able to: • Recognize the essential elements of the medical profession, including moral and ethical principles and legal responsibilities underlying the profession; • Demonstrate professional values which include excellence, responsibility, compassion, empathy, accountability, honesty and integrity, and a commitment to scientific methods.	Introduction to medicine modules. • Hospital visit • PHC unite visit	• Role modelling • Interactive Lectures • SGS • WGS • Hospital visits • PHC wkly	

	• Show respect for patients, peers, faculty and other health professionals to foster a positive learning collaboration with them. • Demonstrate accountability to patients, society and profession, and a commitment to excellence and on-going professional development. • Demonstrate self-regulation and recognition of the need for continuous self-improvement. • Exhibit the ability to effectively plan and efficiently manage one's own time.			• Written exam • PRRE • 360º(Faculty observation and feedback)
6. Population health and health system	Student will be able to: • Explain important life-style, genetic, demographic, environmental, social, economic, psychological, and cultural determinants of the specific system disease at a population level. • Describe the important determinants and risk factors of health & illness, interaction between man and his physical and social environment.	Introduction to medicine modules. • Hospital visit • PHC unite visit	• Interactive Lectures • WGS • Hospital and PHC weekly Visits • E-learning • Mentorship • Self-Directed Learning	• Written exam • PRRE • 360º(Faculty observation and feedback)
7. Management of information	Student will be able to: • Practice searching and interpreting health and biomedical information relevant to understanding health and illnesses. • Integrate information and communication technology to assist in learning.	Hospital visit Weekly primary health care unit visit	• Interactive Lectures • E-learning • Self-Directed Learning	• Student presentation • 360º(Faculty feedback and observation) • OSPE • PRRE

Preclinical Courses (Introductory Block)
Course Description

Preclinical courses are also referred to as the introductory block or the introductory module. The primary objective of the introductory block of the program is to offer a general overview of biomedical sciences prior to the integrated system based blocks. The student will study the general structure, function, biological mechanisms governing homeostasis, the genetic, biochemical, physiologic, and pathologic mechanisms underlying disease states, classification of micro-organisms, host defence and immunology, mechanisms of drug action, pharmacokinetics, pharmacy-dynamics and therapeutics. This will be complemented by longitudinal courses of professional competency development (PCD): history of medicine (International and national), traditional medicine (in context country) and social and population health (SPH) courses: Introduction to determinants of health and health care advocacy.

Course Design

These courses will be given during the first sixteen weeks of Year 1 for the student can gain a general overview of biomedical sciences along with the professional competency development (PCD) and social and population health (SPH) components. The student will also receive orientation to the different teaching and learning methods of the program at this time

Module / Block Objective

To offer the student a general overview of biomedical sciences prior to the integrated system based blocks of the program. The student will study the general structure, function, biological mechanisms governing homeostasis, the genetic, biochemical, physiologic, and pathologic mechanisms underlying disease states, classification of micro-organisms, host defence and immunology, mechanisms of drug action, pharmacokinetics, pharmacy-dynamics and therapeutics.

Section I

Biomedical Sciences

This section is divided into two parts:

1. Section **IA** is a guide to classroom teaching and learning.
2. Section **IB** is a guide to integrated biomedical laboratory and practice.

Section IA

Biomedical Sciences
Classroom Learning

This section provides a guide with a focus to (but not limited) structured classroom learning. It includes the following courses:

1. Anatomy
2. Histology
3. Embryology
4. Physiology
5. Biochemistry
6. Pathology
7. Microbiology
8. Immunology
9. Pharmacology

Anatomy

Course / Subject: Anatomy	
Course / Subject Time Distribution: Lecture - 30 Hours PBL – 6 IL - 24 Hours WGS - 7 Hours	
Course Objectives	By the end of this course the student is expected: 1. To identify and explain the different divisions of anatomy 2. To define descriptive terms and different body movements in anatomy including terms of position and relation 3. To describe the nature and organization of the major, grossly visible structural components of the dissected human body
Course Content	1. The different divisions of anatomy: general anatomy, special anatomy, gross or macroscopic anatomy, 2. Descriptive terms in anatomy including terms of position and relation. 3. The different body movements: axes of movement (longitudinal, sagittal, transverse or horizontal), movements-lateral and medial rotation, flexion and extension, abduction and adduction, circumduction, 4. Names of the bones of the body and their position; classification of the bones, general features of the bone, classification and identification of the muscles of the body: main attachments, nerve supply and action, details of attachments of the muscles, 5. Mechanism of the movement caused by the muscle/muscles and various forces exerted by them and their detailed action(s). 6. Definition and classification of joints, general features of different types of joints; detailed study of major joints of the limbs and movements performed at various joints in the body; blood supply nerve supply.
Training Exercises	Integrated with the practical based lectures: • Visit laboratories for practicals to complement classroom activities • Computer based simulations of gross anatomy may be used for individual or group study. This can be a repetitive reference as need be for deeper processing of concepts. • Prepare lecture and hand-outs for the relevant topics to be presented. • Encourage the student to research on topics prior to the lesson so that the lesson reinforces already learnt material or informative discussions can be held with the class or trainer

	• Models / skeletons provide an opportunity for the student to manipulate the bones to enhance understanding of all the features described in theory. • Computer based learning materials including videos / VCDs can be developed for continuous revision, reflection and conceptualisation of the topic.
Measurement based on Module Objectives	You may choose to use any or all of the following: • Research reports • Assignments • Small group / whole group presentations • Written tests / skill demonstrations • Journals: Encourage the student to keep a weekly or monthly journal or course-based journal to enable him/her correlate all concepts which build into medicine. • Portfolios: Encourage the student to store all experiences (both successes and failures and make a continuous reflection on the topic). • Summative assessments will be done at the end of the topic or module or semester.
Relevance to Course to other modules or Practice	• To offer the student a general overview of the biomedical sciences along with the professional competency development (PCD) and social and Population Health components. • Complemented by longitudinal courses of professional competency development (PCD): history of medicine (International and national) and traditional medicine in Context country. Social and population health (SPH) courses: Introduction to determinants of health and health care advocacy.
Student Hand-outs	• Provide hand-outs based on lecture notes, your research, audio-visual materials • Provide hand-outs compiled from collaborative and group work presentations • Individual research and case reports may also be compiled for class references.
Audio-Visual Materials / Special Equipment / Resources Required	You may choose to use any or all of the following: • Multimedia equipment including: Computer, LCD projector, Video, VCDs, DVDs, CD- ROMs • White board with white board marker or available resource • Models / skeletons / manikins • Hospital wards • Classroom or anatomy labs • Paper and hand-outs

Reference Materials	1. Moore, K. and A. Agur. *Essential Clinical Anatomy.* 3rd edition, 2007. Lippincott, Williams & Wilkins.
	2. Snell, R. *Clinical Anatomy by Regions.* 8th edition, 2008. Lippincott, Williams & Wilkins. Good presentation of clinical case problems at the end of chapters.
	3. Rohen, J. et al. *Color Atlas of Anatomy.* 7th edition, 2011. Lippincott, Williams & Wilkins.
	4. Netter, F. *Atlas of Human Anatomy.* 4th edition, 2006. Icon Learning Systems.
	5. Standring, S. *Gray's Anatomy: The Anatomical Basis of Clinical Practice.* 40th edition, 2010. Churchill Livingstone.
	6. Moses, K. et al. *Atlas of Clinical Gross Anatomy.* 1st edition, 2005. Mosby-Yearbook.

Histology

Course / Subject: Histology
Course / Subject Time Distribution: Lectures – 10 Hours SGS – 2Hours IL - 8 Hours WGS - 1 Hour

Course Objectives	By the end of this course the student is expected: 1. To illustrate the structure and basic parts (nucleus and cytoplasm) of a cell. 2. To identify and explain the different types of tissues & glands. 3. To describe the standard procedures in the preparation of histological specimen 4. To identify different types of commonly used histological stains.

Course Content	1. **Introduction** (1hr)
	  a) Histology & Its Methods of Study
	    – Standard procedures in the preparation of histological specimen - tissue sampling, fixation, dehydration, clearing, embedding, cutting, staining, mounting
	    – Common histological stains - hematoxylin and eosin, AZAN, Van Gieson, resorcin and fuchsin, nuclear fast red, silver impregnation, iron hematoxylin
	    – Histochemistry - Sudan III and IV, Sudan black, Perl's or Purssian blue reaction, PAS-reaction, Alcian blue reaction, Best carmine stain, Feulgen reaction
	    – Immun- histochemistry
	    – Cell fractionation

	– Methods for direct observation of tissues (exterioration and trans-illumination, transparent chamber method, cell and tissue culture, mechanical micromanipulation, radiation probes, vital staining).
	  b) Types and use of Microscopy
	
	2. **The Cell (3 ½ hrs Total)**
	  c) The Cell Cytoplasm(1 1/2hr)
	    – Cytoplasmic Organelles
	    – Cell membrane
	    – Cell membrane & Mitochondria, & case study
	    – Endoplasmic reticulum (R.E.R + S.E.R)
	    – Golgi apparatus
	    – Lysosomes & case study
	    – Ribosomes & protein synthesis
	    – Cytoskeleton
	    – Centrioles & Cilia

d) The Cell Nucleus (1/2hr)
  – Function & nucleic Acid
  – Components of the nucleus
  – Components nucleolus
e) Biological compounds (1/2hr)
  – Stored food
    o Glycogen
    o Lipid
  – Pigments
    o blood Pigments
    o Melanin
    o Lipofuscin
f) The cell cycle (1/2hr)
  – Cell cycle, cell renewal its various phases, endomitosis, amitosis, ageing and death of cells
  – Stem cell
  – Mitosis
  – Meiosis
g) Chromosomes (1/2hr)
  – Structure & types
  – Sex Chromosome
  – Chromosomal anomalies

3. **Epithelial Tissue (2hrs total)**
a) Cell Layers
  – Simple (one layer)
  – Pseudostratified
  – Stratified (two or more layers)
b) Epithelial cell types
  – Simple
  – Squamous
  – Cuboidal
  – Columnar
c) Pseudostratified
  – layers of cells with nuclei at different levels; not all cells reach surface but all adhere to basal lamina
  – Stratified
  – Squamous keratinized (dry)
  – Squamous nonkeratinized (moist)
  – Cuboidal
  – Transitional
  – Columnar

	4. Connective Tissue & supportive tissue (3 1/2 hrs Total) – Connective tissue cells and intercellular substance (20 min) – Components of the intercellular substance (20 min) – Functions of ground substance, (20 min) – Fixed connective tissue cells, (20 min) – Free connective tissue cell, (20 min) – Structure of the intercellular substance and connective tissue fibres (reticular fibres, collagen fibres, elastic fibres), (20 min) – Types of connective tissue (reticular connective tissue, fatty tissue, fibrous connective tissue or connective tissue proper, loose connective tissue, dense connective tissue), (20 min) – Defence functions of connective tissue (specific and unspecific), (20 min) – Cartilaginous tissue (types of cartilage - hyaline, elastic, fibrous), (20 min) – Bony tissue (basic structure, types of bony tissue, osteoclasts, bone marrow, periosteum and endosteum) (20 min)
Small Group Session Discussion Topics (2 hr)	1. Epithelial Tissue 2. Connective Tissue & supportive tissue
Whole Group Sessions (1hr)	1. Connective Tissue & supportive tissue
Training Exercises	1. Visit Histology labs to complement lectures and print reading materials. 2. Prepare and provide slides. 3. Computer-based simulations of histology may be used for individual or group study. This can be repetitive reference as need be for better understanding of concepts. 4. Prepare lecture and hand-outs for the relevant topics to be presented. 5. Computer-based learning materials; Slides / DVDs / VCDs can be stored for continuous revision and conceptualisation of the topic. 6. The student is encouraged to read on topic prior to the lesson so that the lesson reinforces already learnt material or informative discussions can be held with the class or trainer
Measurement based on Module Objectives	You may choose to use any or all of the following: • Research reports • Assignments • Small group / whole group presentations • Written tests

	• Journals: Encourage the student to keep a weekly or monthly journal or course-based journal to enable him/her correlate all concepts which build into medicine. • Portfolios: Encourage the student to store all experiences (both successes and failures and make a continuous reflection on the topic). • Summative assessments will be done at the end of the topic or module or semester.
Relevance to Course to other modules or Practice	• To offer the student a general overview of the biomedical sciences along with the professional competency development (PCD) and social and Population Health components. • Complemented by longitudinal courses of professional competency development (PCD): history of medicine (International and national) and traditional medicine in Context country. Social and population health (SPH) courses: Introduction to determinants of health and health care advocacy.
Student Hand-outs	• Provide hand-outs based on lecture notes, your research, audio-visual materials • Provide hand-outs compiled from collaborative and group work presentations • Individual research and case reports may also be compiled for class references.
Audio-Visual Materials / Special Equipment / Resources Required	You may choose to use any or all of the following: • Multimedia equipment including: Computer, LCD projector, Video, VCDs, DVDs, CD- ROMs • White board with white board marker or any other resource • Internet • Classroom or histology labs • Paper and hand-outs
Reference Materials	**Histology Textbooks.** 1. McKenzie, J.C. and R.M. Klein, Basic Concepts in Cell Biology and Histology, 2000, McGraw-Hill. ISBN:978-0070369306 2. Kierszenbaum, A. *Histology and Cell Biology: An Introduction to Pathology.* 2nd edition, 2007. Mosby-Yearbook. Very dry style. Includes extensive correlates with biochemistry/cell biology/pathology. 3. Ross, M. & W. Pawlina. *Histology: A Text and Atlas with Correlated Cell and Molecular Biology.* 5th revised edition, 2006. Lippincott, Williams & Wilkins. 4. Stevens, A. and J. Lowe. *Human Histology.* 3rd edition, 2005. Mosby-Yearbook. Concise, with only minimal physiology but with some illustrative pathology.

5. Young, B. et al. *Wheater's Functional Histology: A Text and Colour Atlas.* 5th edition, 2006. Churchill Livingstone. $80. Emphasizes tissue function as well as structure.
6. Telser, A. G. et al. *Elsevier's Integrated Histology.* 2007. Mosby-Elsevier. Concise, includes cross-references to other disciplines.

Histology Atlases.
1. Ross, M., W. Pawlina, and T. Barnash. *Atlas of Descriptive Histology.* 1st edition, 2009.
2. Sinauer Associates, Inc. Highly recommended, provides an extensive set of excellent color micrographs.
3. Rhodin, J. *An Atlas of Histology.* 1976 edition. Oxford University Press.
4. Berman, I. *Color Atlas of Basic Histology.* 3rd edition, 2003. Appleton-Lange.
5. Milikowski, C. & I. Berman. *Color Atlas of Basic Histopathology.* 1st edition, 1997. Appleton-Lange. An excellent resource for images of pathologies.
6. Gartner, L. & J. Hiatt. *Color Atlas of Histology.* 5th edition, 2009. Lippincott, Williams & Wilkins.

7. Schechter & Wood. *Ultrastructure: An Interactive Virtual Electron Microscope.* 2005. Sinauer. $46. Like the out-of-print atlas by Rhodin (above), a laptop running this CD might be used alongside your light microscope as if it were an "extra-high power" objective.
8. Mills, S. *Histology for Pathologists.* 3rd edition, 2007. Lippincott, Williams & Wilkins. $269. Or 2nd edition, 1998, by Sternberg. This text is an excellent, highly recommended reference for details of normal histology beyond what is typically included in introductory textbooks.
9. Kumar, V. et al. *Robbins & Cotran's Pathologic Basis of Disease.* 8th edition, 2009. W. B. Saunders.

Embryology

Course / Subject: Embryology	
Course / Subject Time Distribution: Lecture - 7 Hours PBL / SGS - 1 Hour IL - 4 Hours WGS - 2 Hours	
Course Objectives	By the end of this course the student is expected: 1. To describe basic human embryologic development 2. To describe intrauterine developmental anatomy of the human embryo including the common embryonic anomalies from conception to organogenesis.
Course Content	1. Important terms in embryology (Readings by the student) 2. Gametogenesis (oogenesis, menstrual cycle & spermatogenesis) (1hr) 3. Fertilization, including changes to the endometrium, ovulation &ejaculation (1/2hr) 4. Preimplantation and implantation (1/2hr) 5. Embryonic disk (1hr) 6. Embryonic phase or period of embryogenesis (1hr) 7. The ectoderm, endoderm, and mesoderm and which organ systems arise from them 8. The development of the different organ systems: cardiovascular, respiratory, musculoskeletal, neurologic, renal, gastrointestinal, musculoskeletal, integumentary and endocrine 9. Foetal phase (1hr) 10. Organ maturation 11. Sexual differentiation
	12. Foetal membrane and placenta (1/2hr) 13. The physiologic changes associated with delivery of the foetus. (1/2hr) 14. Chromosomal and gene aberrations and testing(1/2hr) 15. Intrauterine developmental anatomy of the human embryo including the common embryonic anomalies from conception to organogenesis. (1/2hr)
Small Group Session Discussion Topics (1 hr)	1. Embryonic phase or period of embryogenesis (1hr) • The ectoderm, endoderm, and mesoderm and which organ systems arise from them • The development of the different organ systems: cardiovascular, respiratory, musculoskeletal, neurologic, renal, gastrointestinal, musculoskeletal, integumentary and endocrine.

Whole Group Sessions (2 hr)	1. Gametogenesis (oogenesis, menstrual cycle & spermatogenesis) (1hr) 2. Embryonic phase or period of embryogenesis (1hr) • The ectoderm, endoderm, and mesoderm and which organ systems arise from them • The development of the different organ systems: cardiovascular, respiratory, musculoskeletal, neurologic, renal, gastrointestinal, musculoskeletal, integumentary and endocrine 3. Foetal membrane and placenta (1/2hr)
Training Exercises	1. Prepare lecture and hand-outs for the relevant topics to be presented. 2. The student is encouraged to research on topic prior to the lesson so that the lesson reinforces already learnt material or informative discussions can be held with the class or trainer. 3. Models provide an opportunity for the student to manipulate materials to enhance understanding of the features in embryology described in theory. 4. Attend embryology labs (DVD/VCD) to visualise the developmental anatomy of the human embryo. 5. MCH clinic or labour ward in the (health centre) visit for student to interact with mothers to conceptualise the processes of intrauterine development. (Coordinate with SPH) 6. Embryology video / DVD/ VCDs / computer based simulations may be used for individual or group study and for reference and repetitions as need be. Computer Based learning materials e.g. internet sites and videos can be stored for continuous revision and conceptualisation of the topic.
	7. Selected topics will be discussed in small group sessions and whole group sessions to enhance communication and problem solving skills. 8. Advice the student to research on topic prior to the lesson so that the lesson reinforces informative discussions during class.
Measurement based on Module Objectives	You may choose to use any or all of the following: • Small group / whole group presentations • Assignments • Research / case reports • Written tests • Portfolios: student are encouraged to store all experiences (both successes and failures and make a continuous reflection on the topic) • Summative assessments will be done at the end of the topic or module or semester.

Relevance to Course to other modules or Practice	• To offer the student a general overview of the biomedical sciences along with the professional competency development (PCD) and social and Population Health components. • Complemented by longitudinal courses of professional competency development (PCD): history of medicine (International and national) and traditional medicine in Context country. Social and population health (SPH) courses: Introduction to determinants of health and health care advocacy.
Student Hand-outs	• Provide hand-outs based on lecture notes, your research, and audio-visual materials. • Provide hand-outs compiled from collaborative and group work presentations. • Individual research reports may also be compiled for class references.
Audio-Visual Materials / Special Equipment / Resources Required	• Multimedia equipment including: computer, LCD projector, Video, VCDs, DVDs, CD- ROMs • White board with white board marker or available resource • Paper and hand-outs • Models and simulations • MCH clinic or Labour ward • Classroom / integrated laboratories
Reference Materials	1. Moore, K. and T. Persaud. *The Developing Human: Clinically Oriented Embryology.* 8th edition, 2008. Saunders. 2. Sadler, T. W. *Langman's Medical Embryology.* 11th edition, 2009. Lippincott, Williams & Wilkins.

Physiology

Course / Subject: Physiology	
Course / Subject Time Distribution: Lectures - 30 Hours SGS - 5 Hours IL - 12 Hours WGS - 8 Hours	
Course Objectives	By the end of this course the student is expected: 1. To outline the overview of human physiology and prepare the student for system based physiology. 2. To illustrate how the different components of the human cell contribute towards its function. 3. To describe and explain homeostasis & regulation in the human body. 4. To explain the basics of DNA & RNA synthesis, membrane, nerve and muscle physiology.

Course Content	**1) Introduction to physiology (Time alloted 15 min)**
	   a) Introduction, history, goal & objectives
	2) Functional Organization of the Human Body and Control of the "Internal Environment":
	   a) The cell,
	   b) Intracellular and extracellurla fluid,
	   c) Homeostatic and control systems of the body
	   1. Cells as the living units of the body (2hr)
	   a) Illustrate the structure and basic parts (nucleus and cytoplasm) of a cell. Illustrate the structure and function of cell membrane.
	      i. Organization of the cell
	      ii. Membranous structures of the cell
	      iii. Cytoplasm and its organelles
	      iv. Nucleus
	      v. Nuclear membrane
	      vi. Nucleoli and formation of ribosomes
	      vii. Functional systems of the cell
	         a) Ingestion by the cell-endocytosis
	         b) Digestion of pinocytotic and phagocytic foreign substances inside the cell-function of the lysosomes
	         c) Synthesis and formation of cellular structures by endoplasmic reticulum and golgi apparatus
	         d) Extraction of energy from nutrients-function of the mitochondria
	   2. Extracellular Fluid- the "Internal Environment" (1/2hr)

3. "Homeostatic" Mechanisms of the Major Functional Systems
   i. Homeostasis & Regulation
     a) Intrinsic control mechanisms of the organism
     b) Regulatory principles in physiology (1hr)
        – Problem of the norm & normal range
        – Control theory
        – single loop feedback system
        – Multiple loop feedback system+
        – Negative feedback
        – Positive feedback
        – Stability & oscillations
  ii. Control systems and regulation of body functions (examples) (30min)
     a) Nervous system.
     b) Hormonal system of regulation
     c) Regulation of oxygen and carbon dioxide concentrations in the extracellular fluid.
     d) Regulation of arterial blood pressure
 iii. Extracellular fluid (60min)
     a) Transport and mixing system-the blood circulatory system
     b) Normal ranges and physical characteristics of important extracellular fluid constituents
 iv. Origin of nutrients in the extracellular fluid: (reading for student)(30min)
  v. Removal of metabolic end products: (reading for student)
     a) Lungs: removal of carbon dioxide.
     b) Kidneys: removal of **urea** and uric acid;
     c) Skin

3) The Cell and its functions: Genes, DNA, RNA
  a. Genes in the cell nucleus (30min)
     i. Genetic code
  b. The DNA code in the cell nucleus is transferred to an RNA code in the cell cytoplasm
     i. The process of transcription (2hrs)
     ii. Synthesis of RNA
     iii. Assembly of the RNA chain from activated nucleotides using the DNA strand as a template-the process of "transcription"

      iv. Messenger RNA-the codons

      v. Transfer RNA-the anticodons

      vi. Ribosomal RNA

      vii. Formation of proteins on the ribosomes-the process of "translation"

  c. Synthesis of other substances in the cell (20min)

  d. Control of gene function and biochemical activity in cells (3hr)

      i. Genetic regulation

      ii. Control of intracellular function by enzyme regulation

      iii. The DNA-genetic system also controls cell reproduction

        a) Cell reproduction begins with replication of DNA

        b) Chromosomes and their replication

        c) Cell mitosis

        d) Control of cell growth and cell reproduction

  e. Cell differentiation (15min)

  f. Apoptosis-programmed cell death (15min)

  g. Cancer (30hr)

4) Nerve and membrane physiology

  a. The plasma membrane (1hr)

      i. The Lipid bi-layer

      ii. Membrane proteins; types, functions

      iii. Membrane transport of small molecules

      iv. Diffusion, active transport

      v. Membrane transport of macromolecules & particles

  b. Cell signalling (control of cell function) (1hr)

      i. Cell signalling by electrical excitation

      ii. Membrane potential

        – Potential & ionic pypotheis

        – Electrotonus & passive electrical properties of membrane

        – Measurement of membrane potential

  c. Action Potential (1hr)

      i. Initiation of AP

      ii. Behavior of ionic channels in AP

      iii. Stimulus parameters

      iv. All -or- none principle & refractoriness

      v. Propagation of AP

d. Special characteristics of signal transmission in nerve trunks (1hr)

    i. Brief anatomy of the nerve

    ii. Myelinated and unmyelinated nerve fibers.

    iii. "Saltatory" conduction in myelinated fibers from node to node.

    iv. Velocity of conduction in nerve fibers.

    v. Excitation-the process of eliciting the action potential

e. Transmission of excitation from cell-to cell/synapses (1hr)

    i. Chemical synaptic transmission

    ii. Synaptic receptors

    iii. Synaptic transmitter

    iv. Types of synapses / inhibitory / excitatory

    v. Synaptic potentials

    vi. Integration of synaptic events

    vii. Electrical synaptic transmission

    viii. Cross talks between nerves

f. Cell communication by autacoid and paracrine hormones (2hrs)

    i. Introduction; endocrine, paracrine & autocrine control

    ii. Prostaglandins, thromboxanes & leukotrienes

    iii. Cytokines:

       – Overview

       – Individual cytokines & their properties

       – The cytokine network

    iv. Nitric oxide & other endothelial derived factors

    v. Bradykinin, histamine, serotonin, platelet activating factor

       – The kallikrin-kinin system

       – Histamine & serotoin

       – Platelet activating factor

g. Cellular transduction process (3hrs)

    i. Introduction

    ii. The CAMP cascade & phosphorylation

    iii. Inositol- triphosphate

    iv. Diacyl glycerol

    v. Calcium as a second messenger

    vi. Calcium influx, calcium release, calcium store and uptake, calcium stores & their regulation, calcium binding proteins

    vii. Cyclic GMP

    viii. RAS proteins & other GTP- binding proteins

	5) Physiology of muscle cell
	  a. Functional structure of the skeletal muscle (30min)
	  b. Molecular bases of contraction (1 hr)
	    i. The contractile proteins (actin, myosin, tropomyosin, troponin)
	    ii. Cross bridge activity
	    iii. Sliding filament theory
	    iv. Mode of action of ATP
	  c. Muscle excitation(hr)
	    i. Neuromuscular junction (30min)
	    ii. Motor unit (30min)
	    iii. Excitation contraction coupling (30min)
	    iv. Muscle mechanics (1hr)
	      – Mechanical properties of resting muscle
	      – Isotonic & Isometric contractions
	      – Length - tension relation
	      – Load-shortening relation
	      – Force-Velocity relation
	      – single twitch, superposition & tetanus
	      – Muscle force control
	      – Recruitment tetanization & fatigue
	      – Elastic element of force of contraction
	      – Musculo-skeletal mechanics
	      – Muscle force & excitability
	    v. Muscle energetics (1hr)
	      – Energy metabolism
	      – Fatigue & recovery
	      – Muscle heat & energy turnover
	      – Efficiency & work out put
	      – Metabolic subtypes of muscle fibers
	      – Remolding of muscle
	    vi. Smooth muscle cell (1hr)
	      – Comparison with skeletal muscle
	      – control of smooth muscles contraction (neuronal, humeral, miscellaneous)
	      – MP & AP in smooth muscles
	      – Plasticity
	    vii. Overview of cardiac muscle(1hr)

Small Group Session Discussion Topics (5 hours)	1. Extracellular fluid-the "internal environment" 2. DNA synthesis 3. RNA synthesis 4. Membrane physiology and signaling 5. Special characteristics of signal transmission in nerve trunks

Whole Group Sessions (8 hours)	1. Cells as the living units of the body 2. Extracellular fluid-the "internal environment" 3. "Homeostatic" mechanisms of the major functional systems 4. DNA synthesis 5. RNA synthesis 6. Membrane physiology and signaling 7. Special characteristics of signal transmission in nerve trunks 8. Function and structure of the skeletal muscle
Training Exercises	• Prepare lecture and hand-outs for the topics to be presented. • Integrated laboratories to conceptualise human physiology. • The student is encouraged to research on topic prior to the lesson so that the lesson reinforces already learnt material or informative discussions can be held within the class on **small group sessions and whole group sessions** with you. • DVD / VCDs / computer based simulations may be used for individual or group study and for reference and repetitions as need be. • Computer-based learning materials e.g. internet sites and videos can be stored for continuous revision and conceptualisation of the topic
Measurement based on Module Objectives	The trainer may choose to use any or all of the following: • Small group / whole group presentations • Assignments • Research / case reports • Written tests • Journals: Encourage the student to keep a weekly or monthly journal or course-based journal to enable him/her correlate all concepts which build into medicine. • Portfolios: Encourage the student to store all experiences (both successes and failures and make a continuous reflection on the topic). • Summative assessments will be done at the end of the topic or module or semester.
Relevance to Course to other modules or Practice	• To offer the student a general overview of the biomedical sciences along with the professional competency development (PCD) and social and Population Health components. • Complemented by longitudinal courses of professional competency development (PCD): history of medicine (International and national) and traditional medicine in Context country. Social and population health (SPH) courses: Introduction to determinants of health and health care advocacy.

Student Hand-outs	• Provide hand-outs based on lecture notes, Trainer's research, audio-visual materials • Provide hand-outs compiled from collaborative and group work presentations. • Individual research reports may also be compiled for class references. • Case presentation reports may also be compiled for class references.
Audio-Visual Materials / Special Equipment / Resources Required	You may choose to use any or all of the following: • Classroom or integrated lab • Paper and Hand-outs • Multimedia equipment including: computer, LCD projector, Video, VCDs, DVDs, CD- ROMs • White board with white board marker or available resource
Reference Materials	1. Guyton and Hall, Textbook of Medical Physiology, 12th Edition 2. Vander's Human Physiology: The Mechanisms of Body Function

Biochemistry

Course / Subject: Biochemistry	
Course / Subject Time Distribution: Lectures - 23 Hours PBL - 4 Hours IL - 8 Hours WGS - 10 Hours	
Course Objectives	By the end of this course the student is expected: 1. To analyze the body fluid buffer systems 2. To classify and define different forms of metabolism. 3. To describe principles of biological catalysis and application of enzymology in diagnosis and drug mechanism of action 4. To explain principles of genetic information storage and expression
Course Content	1. The body fluid buffer systems, different forms of metabolism, the principles of biological catalysis and application of enzymology in diagnosis and drug mechanism of action. 2. Function and classification of carbohydrates, lipids, protein and amino acids. 3. Stereoisomerism and chemistry of monosaccharides, amino acids, and fatty acids. 4. Structural organization and structure-function relationships of proteins. Hemoglobin and myoglobin, 5. Pathways of glucose metabolism: glycolysis, HMP shunt, Krebs cycle gluconeogenesis, glycogenolysis, glycogenesis, biosynthesis and degradation of fatty acids, phospolipids and triacylglycerols, biosynthesis of cholesterol, chemistry and metabolism of lipoproteins.
	6. Molecular basis of hormonal action, signal transduction mechanisms. – Nucleic acids: DNA and RNA structure – DNA replication, – DNA transcription – Post-transcriptional processing. – Translation of genetic code – Regulation of gene expression and protein synthesis inhibitors of protein synthesis. – DNA repair mechanisms,
Training Exercises	• Integrate lectures with lab experience. • Experiential learning • Prepare lecture and hand-outs for the relevant topics to be presented. • The student is encouraged to research on topic prior to the lesson so that the lesson reinforces already learnt material or informative discussions can be held with the class or trainer.

	• Computer-based learning materials, videos, VCDs, WWW, can be used for continuous revision and conceptualisation of the topic.
Measurement based on Module Objectives	You may choose to use any or all of the following: • Research reports • Assignments • Small group / whole group presentations • Written tests • Journals: Encourage the student to keep a weekly or monthly journal or course-based journal to enable him/her correlate all concepts which build into medicine. • Portfolios: Encourage the student to store all experiences (both successes and failures and make a continuous reflection on the topic). • Summative assessments will be done at the end of the topic or module or semester.
Relevance to Course to other modules or Practice	• To offer the student a general overview of the biomedical sciences along with the professional competency development (PCD) and social and Population Health components. • Complemented by longitudinal courses of professional competency development (PCD): history of medicine (International and national) and traditional medicine in Context country. Social and population health (SPH) courses: Introduction to determinants of health and health care advocacy.
Student Hand-outs	• Provide hand-outs based on lecture notes, your research, audio-visual materials • Provide hand-outs compiled from collaborative and group work presentations • Individual research reports may also be compiled for class references. • Case presentation reports may also be compiled for class references.
Audio-Visual Materials / Special Equipment / Resources Required	You may choose to use any or all of the following: • Multimedia equipment including: computer, LCD projector, Video, VCDs, DVDs, and CD- ROMs. • White board with white board marker or available resource • paper and Hand-outs • Models • Hospital wards • Classroom / Lab

Reference Materials	1. Lehninger Principles of Biochemistry (5th Ed) David L. Nelson and Michael M. Cox - ISBN13:9780716771081
	2. Berg, J.M., Stryer, L, Tymoczko, J.L., Biochemistry, 6th Ed., Freeman, W. H. & Company
	3. Lieberman, M. A. and A. Marks. *Marks' Essential Medical Biochemistry: A Clinical Approach.* 3rd edition, 2009. Lippincott, Williams & Wilkins.
	4. Biochemistry (6th Ed) Jeremy M. Berg, John L. Tymoczko & Lubert Stryer – IBN13:9780716787242
	5. Salway, J. *Medical Biochemistry at a Glance.* 2nd edition, 2006. Blackwell. $39. A good overview with pertinent details and illustrations.
	6. Devlin, T. *Textbook of Biochemistry with Clinical Correlations.* 7th edition, 2010. John Wiley & Sons. $192. comprehensive reference book ISBN-13: 978-0470281734
	7. Murray, R. K., D. K. Granner, and V. W. Rodwell. *Harper's Illustrated Biochemistry.* 28th edition, 2009. McGraw Hill. $55.
	8. Berg, J.M., Stryer, L, Tymoczko, J.L., Biochemistry, 6th Ed., Freeman, W. H. & Company
	9. Champe, P.C. et al. *Biochemistry: Lippincott's Illustrated Reviews.* 4th edition, 2008. Lippincott, Williams & Wilkins.
	10. McGilvery, Robert W. Biochemistry, a Functional Approach. 2d ed. Philadelphia, Saunders,1979.

Pathology

Course / Subject: Pathology
Course / Subject Time Distribution: Lecture - 25 Hours PBL - 5 Hours IL - 13 Hours WGS - 8 Hours

Course Objectives	By the end of this course the student is expected: 1. To explain the mechanisms of cell injury and death 2. To describe the process of wound healing and repair 3. To define inflammation and enumerate its cardinal signs Classify neoplasia and explain molecular basis of cancer including cellular interaction of carcinogenic agents of genetic information storage and expression.

Course Content	**1. Cell injury, adaptation and death**
	  a) Introduction to pathology (1/4hr)
	  b) Overview of cell injury
	    1. Causes of cell injury(1/2hr)
	      – Oxygen deprivation.
	      – Chemical agents.
	      – Infectious agents.
	      – Immunologic reactions
	    2. Mechanisms of cell injury (1/2hr)
	      – General biochemical mechanisms
	      – Ischemic and hypoxic injury
	      – Ischemia / reperfusion injury
	      – Free radical-induced cell injury
	      – Chemical injury
	    3. Cellular adaptation to injury (1hr)
	      – Atrophy
	      – Hypertrophy
	      – Hyperplasia
	      – Metaplasia
	      – Subcellular responses to injury
	      – Intracellular accumulations
	      – Pathologic calcification
	    4. Reversible and irreversible cell injury(1/2hr)
	      1. General pathways
	      2. Mechanisms of irreversible injury
	      3. Morphology of reversible cell injury and cell death-necrosis
	    5. Programmed cell death-apoptosis (1/4hr)
	    6. Cellular aging(1/4hr)

2. General pathology of infectious diseases
   a) History / new and emerging infectious diseases (1/4hr)
   b) Categories of infectious agents (1/4hr) Relate to Microbiology
   c) Host barriers to infection and how they break down(1/4hr)
      1. Skin
      2. Urogenital tract
      3. intestinal tract
   d) Spread of microbes throughout the body (1/4hrRelate to Microbiology
      1. Release of microbes from the body
   e) How infectious agents cause disease (1/4hr) Relate to Microbiology
      1. Mechanisms of virus-induced injury
      2. Mechanisms of bacteria-induced injury: bacterial adhesions and toxins
      3. Immune evasion by microbes (1/4hr) Relate to Immunology

3. Acute and chronic inflammation
   a) Overview of inflammation(1/4hr)
   b) Acute inflammation(1hr)
      1. Cellular events
      2. Defects in leukocyte function
      3. Chemical mediators of inflammation
      4. inflammation-induced tissue injury
      5. outcomes of acute inflammation
   c) Chronic inflammation(1hr)
      1. Chronic inflammatory cells and mediators
      2. Granulomatous inflammation
      3. Lymphatics and lymph nodes in inflammation
   d) Systemic effects of inflammation (1/2hr)
   e) Inflammatory response to infectious agents(1/4hr) Relate to Immunology

4. Tissue repair: cell regeneration and fibrosis
   a) Overview of the inflammatory-reparative response(1/4hr)
   b) Cell regeneration (1/2hr)
      1. Control of cell growth and differentiation
      2. Soluble mediators
      3. Extracellular matrix and cell-matrix interactions
   c) Repair by connective tissue (fibrosis) (1/2hr)
      1. Angiogenesis
      2. Fibrosis (scar formation)
      3. Scar remodeling
   d) Growth factors in cell regeneration and fibrosis (1/4hr)

e) Wound healing (1hr)
  1. Healing by second intention
  2. Healing by second intention
  3. Wound strength
f) Pathologic aspects of repair (1/2hr)

5. Hemodynamic disorders, thrombosis, and shock
  1. Edema (1/2hr)
  2. Hyperemia and congestion (1/4hr)
  3. Hemorrhage (1/4hr)
  4. Hemostasis and thrombosis (1/2hr)
     a. Normal hemostasis
     b. Thrombosis
  5. Embolism (1/2hrs)
     a. Pulmonary thromboembolism
     b. Systemic thromboembolism
     c. Fat embolism
     d. Amniotic fluid embolism
  6. Infarction (1/2hr)
  7. Shock (1hr)
     a. Pathogenesis of septic shock
     b. Stages of shock
  8. Diseases of immunity
     a. Cells of the immune system (1/2hr)
        i. T lymphocytes
        ii. B lymphocytes
        iii. Macrophages
        iv. Dendritic cells
        v. Natural killer (nk) cells
     b. Histocompatibility molecules(1/4hr)
     c. Cytokines: soluble mediators of the immune system(1/4hr)
     d. Mechanisms of immune-mediated injury (hypersensitivity reactions) (1/2hr)
        i. Type i hypersensitivity
        ii. Type ii hypersensitivity
        iii. Type iii hypersensitivity
        iv. Type iv hypersensitivity
        v. Transplant rejection
     e. Autoimmune diseases (1/4hr)
     f. Immunodeficiency diseases(1/4hr)
        i. Primary immunodeficiencies
        ii. Secondary immunodeficiencies
        iii. Acquired immunodeficiency syndrome
     g. Amyloidosis ((1/4hr)

6. Neoplasia

  a. Definitions (1/4hr)

  b. Nomenclature(1/4hr)

  c. Characteristics of benign and malignant neoplasms (1hr)

    1. Differentiation and anaplasia

    2. Rate of growth

    3. Local invasion

    4. Metastasis

  d. Epidemiology carcinogenesis (1/4hr)

    1. Cancer incidence

    2. Geographic and environmental factors

    3. Age

    4. Heredity

    5. Acquired preneoplastic disorders

  e. Overview of Carcinogenesis: the molecular basis of cancer(1/2hr)

    1. Self-sufficiency in growth signals

    2. Insensitivity to growth-inhibitory signals

    3. Evasion of apoptosis

    4. Limitless replicative potential

    5. Development of sustained angiogenesis

    6. Ability to invade and metastasize

    7. Genomic instability-enabler of malignancy

    8. Molecular basis of multistep carcinogenesis

    9. Karyotypic changes in tumors

  f. Etiology of cancer: carcinogenic agents(1/2hr)

    1. Chemical carcinogens

    2. Radiation carcinogenesis

    3. Viral and microbial oncogenesis

  g. Host defense against tumors: tumor immunity(1/2hr)

    1. Tumor antigens

    2. Antitumor effector mechanisms

    3. Immunosurveillance

  h. Clinical features of neoplasia(1/2hr)

    1. Effects of tumor on host

    2. Grading and staging of cancer

    3. Laboratory diagnosis of cancer

  i. Genetic and pediatric diseases

    1. Genetic diseases (1/2hr)

      i. Mutations

      ii. Mendelian disorders (diseases caused by single-gene defects)

      iii. Disorders with multifactorial inheritance

	iv. Cytogenetic disorders
	v. Single-gene disorders with atypical patterns of inheritance
	2. Pediatric diseases (1/2hr)
	   i. Congenital anomalies
	   ii. Hydrops fetalis
	   iii. Cystic fibrosis
	3. Diagnosis of genetic diseases (1/4hr)
	j. Environmental diseases
	   1. Environmental pollution (1/4hr)
	     i. Air pollution
	     ii. Industrial exposures
	   2. Tobacco smoke (1/4hr)
	   3. Injury by chemical agents (1/4hr)
	   4. Mechanical trauma (Reading)
	   5. Thermal injury (Reading)
	   6. Electrical injury (Reading)
	   7. Injury produced by ionizing radiation (Reading)

Training Exercises	• Visit pathology/ histology labs to integrate with theory. • You may use videos for individual or group study because it can be rewound or forwarded for better understanding of concepts. • Prepare lecture and hand-outs for the relevant topics to be presented. • Encourage the student to research on the topic prior to the lesson so that the lesson reinforces already learnt material and informative discussions can be held during class. • Case studies may be done at the clinics to enhance contact with actual patients and presented in class to enhance communication and problem solving skills. • Models provide an opportunity for the student to touch the material and practice handling procedures prior to the actual human contact. • Computer Based learning materials like videos can be used for continuous revision and conceptualisation of the topic.
Measurement based on Module Objectives	You may choose to use any or all of the following: • Research reports • Assignments • Small group / whole group presentations • Written tests

	• Journals: Encourage the student to keep a weekly or monthly journal or course-based journal to enable him/her correlate all concepts which build into medicine. • Portfolios: Encourage the student to store all experiences (both successes and failures and make a continuous reflection on the topic). • Summative assessments will be done at the end of the topic or module or semester.
Relevance to Course to other modules or Practice	To offer the student a general overview of the biomedical sciences along with the professional competency development (PCD) and social and Population Health components. Complemented by longitudinal courses of professional competency development (PCD): history of medicine (International and national) and traditional medicine in Context country. Social and population health (SPH) courses: Introduction to determinants of health and health care advocacy.
Student Hand-outs	• Provide hand-outs based on lecture notes, Trainer's research, audio-visual materials • Provide hand-outs compiled from collaborative and group work presentations • Individual research reports may also be compiled for class references. • Case presentation reports may also be compiled for class references.
Audio-Visual Materials / Special Equipment / Resources Required	You may choose to use any or all of the following: • Multimedia equipment including: computer, LCD projector, Video, VCDs, DVDs, CD- ROMs • White board with white board marker or Blackboard with chalk • Models • Wards • Classroom / Lab • Paper and Hand-outs
Reference Materials	1. Robbins, S.L. and Ramzi S. Cotran, Pathological Basis of Disease, 7th Ed., 2005, ElsevierSaunders Inc. 2. Lange Physiology Series, Endocrine Physiology, Molina, 2nd Ed. 3. Kumar V, Abbas A, & Fasto N; Pathologic Basis of Disease, Elsevier-Saunders, 2009. ISBN:0721601871

Microbiology

Course / Subject: Microbiology	
Course / Subject Time Distribution: Lectures - 25 Hours PBL - 4 Hours IL - 15 Hours WGS - 5 Hours	
Course Objectives	By the end of this course the student is expected: 1. To classify microorganisms and illustrate their cellular/anatomic characteristics in general. 2. To explain the process of bacterial growth, multiplication and death including bacterial physiology and nutrition. 3. To identify the different mechanisms of disinfection and sterilization

Course Content	1. Rationale for classifying microbes into bacteria, fungi viruses, parasites
	2. The nature of bacteria
	3. Morphological differences and Growth requirement of bacteria
	4. Nomenclature and classification of bacteria
	5. Biology of protozoa
	6. Medically important helminths
	7. Ectoparasites
	8. The nature and properties of viruses
	9. Brief appraisal of pathogenicity of viruses
	10. Nature of fungi: basic structures and classification
	11. Sterilization and disinfection
	12. Different mechanisms of disinfection and sterilization
	13. General Microbiology
	    a) Introduction to microbiology (1/2hr)
	    b) Important concepts (1hr)
	        i. Structure
	        ii. taxonomy
	        iii. Pathogenesis
	        iv. Host defenses
	        v. epidemiology
	        vi. Laboratory diagnoses
	        vii. Sterilization and disinfection
	        viii. Antibiotic sensitivity testing
	        ix. Unique differentiating features of eukaryotes and prokaryotes
	    c) What is diagnostic microbiology (1hr)
	        i. Tests
	        ii. Microscopes
	        iii. Staining
	        iv. Cell culture
	        v. Cloning

d) **How to approach each pathogen (1hr)**
   i.   Class
   ii. Structure
   iii. Epidemiology Source and spread of microbes
   iv. Mechanism of host entry and pathogenesis
   v.   Host defenses
   vi. Replication
   vii. Sites of dissemination and Clinical presentation
   viii. Diagnostic tests
   ix. Laboratory diagnosis
   x.   Pharmaceutical management and antibiotic resistance pattern

e) **Classification of Microbes: Bacteria, Viruses, Fungi and Parasites**
   i. **Bacteria**
      a) Overview of major pathogens: (2hr)
         i.   Staining: Gram staining, acid fast staining, india ink
         ii. Properties of Gram positive and gram negative organisms
         iii. Using properties to categorize:
            – Coagulase +/-
            – Spore forming
            – Conditions: aerobic, anaerobic, facultative
            – Location of bacteria-intracellular vs. extracellular
            – Shapes: Cocci, rods, coccobacilli, filamentous,
            – Motility: pilli, flagellae
         iv. Adaptations: pilli, endotoxins, exotoxin
      b) Bacterial genetics (1/4hr)
      c) Gram positive cocci (1/2hr)
         – Streptococci-pyogenes, bovis, pneumoniae, mutans, intermedius
         – Staphylococcus-aureus, epidermis, saprophyticus, agalactiae
      d) Gram negative cocci (1/2hr)
         i.   Neisseria-meningitidis, gonorrhoeae
      e) Gram positive bacilli (1/2hr)
         i.   Bacillus-anthacis, cereus
         ii. Clostridium tetani, botulinum, difficile, perfrigens, diptheriae
         iii. Listeriae
         iv. Actinomyces

f) Gram negative bacilli (1hr)
   i. Klebsiella. pneumonia
   ii. Escheri. Coli
   iii. Salmonella-typhi, enteritidis, dysenteriae
   iv. Proteus mirabilis
   v. Vibrio colerae
   vi. Pseudomonas aeruginosa
   vii. Yersinia enterolitica, pestis
   viii. Helicobacter pylori
   ix. Campylobacter jejuni
   x. Bacteroides fragilis

g) Gram negative coccobacilli (1/2hr)
   i. Hemophilus influenza
   ii. Listeriae pneu, ophilia
   iii. Bortella pertussis
   iv. Brucella
   v. Francisemia tularensis

h) Mycobacteria (1hr)
   i. Acid-fast staining
   ii. Mycobacterium tuberculosis
   iii. Mycobacterium leprae
   iv. Atypical Mycobacteriae

i) Actinomycetes(1/2hr)
   i. Actinomyces israelii
   ii. Nocardia asteroides

j) Mycoplasma1/4
   i. Mycoplasma pneumonia
   ii. Mycoplasma hominis

k) Spirochetes(1/2hr)
   i. Diagnostic tests: darkfield microscopy, silver
      impregnation, immunofluorescence
   ii. Shape: flexible, spiral rods
   iii. Motile
   iv. Treponema
   v. Borrelia
   vi. Leptospira

l) Chlamydiae (1/2hr)
   i. C. trachomatis
   ii. C. pneumonia
   iii. C. psittaci

m) Rickettsiae (1/2hr)
   i. R. rickettsii
   ii. R. prowazekii
   iii. Coxiella burnetii

n) Bacterial vaccinations (1/2hr)

ii. Basic virology (1hr)
 a) Classifcation
 b) Structure
 c) Replication: DNA vs. RNA based
 d) Genetics and gene therapy
iii. Clinical virology
 a) DNA-based
  i. DNA enveloped viruses (1hr)
   a. Herpesevirus
    i. Herpes Simplex Virus
    ii. Varicella Zoster Virus
    iii. Cytomegalovirus
    iv. Epstein-Barr Virus
    v. Human Herpesvirus 8
   b. Poxvirus
    i. Smallpox virus
    ii. Molluscum Contagiosum Virus
    iii. Hepatitis B Virus
  ii. DNA nonenveloped viruses (1hr)
   a. Adenovirus
   b. Papillomaviruses
   c. Parvoviruses
   d. Polyomaviruses- JC virus, BK birus
 b) RNA-based
  i. Enveloped viruses (1hr)
   a. Orthomyxoviruses (Influenza viruses)
   b. Paramyxoviruses: Measles, Mumps, Respiratory Syncytial Virus, Parainfluenza viruses
   c. Coronavirus: Coronavirus
   d. Togaviruses: Rubella Virus,
   e. Rhabdoviruses: Rabies virus
   f. Retroviruses: Human T-Cell Lymphotropic Virus
  ii. Nonenveloped viruses (1/2hr)
   a. Picornaviruses: Enteroviruses, Rhinoviruses
   b. Caliciviruses: Caliciviruses, Norwalk virus
   c. Reoviruses: Rotavirus
 c) Hepatic viruses (1hr)
  i. Overview: mechanism of transmission, infect
  ii. Hepatitis A Virus
  iii. Hepatitis B Virus
  iv. Hepatitis C Virus

    v.   Hepatitis D Virus
    vi. Hepatitis E Virus
    vii. Hepatitis G Virus
  d) Human Immunodeficiency Virus (1hr)
     i. Special structural properties
     ii. Retrovirus
     iii. Special genes and proteins
  e) Arboviruses-arthropod-born viruses(1/4hr)
     i. Togaviruses-rubella
     ii. Flaviviruses
     iii. Bunyaviruses
  f) Tumor viruses (1/2hr)
     i. Malignant transformation of cells
     ii. Proviruses and oncogenes (promoting growth factors)
     iii. Vaccinations against cancer: HBV, HPV
  g) Prions (1/4hr)
     i. Structure
     ii. Mechanism of propagation
     iii. Site of attack
     iv. Examples: Kuru, CJD

iv. Mycology
  a) Basics of mycology (1hr)
     i. Classiciation
     ii. Morphology
     iii. Reproduction
     iv. 4 categories: cutaneous, subcutaneous, systemic, and opportunistic
  b) Cutaneous and subcutaneous mycoses (1hr)
     i. Dermatophytes- Epidermophyton, Trichophyton, and microsporum
       a. Tinea capitus, T. corporis. T. cruris, T. pedis
       b. Tinea veriscolor
       c. Tinea Nigra
  c) Systemic mycoses (1hr)
     i. Dimorphic fungi that differentiate into either yeasts or other shapes
     ii. Coccidiodes
     iii. Histoplasma
     iv. Blastomyces
     v. Paracoccidiodes

d) Opportunistic mycoses (1hr)
  i. Which hosts are especially susceptible
  ii. Candida
  iii. Cryptococcus
  iv. Aspergillus
  v. Mucor & Rhizopus
  vi. Pneumocystis

v. Parasitology
  a) Overview-forms (helminthes & protozoa) (1hr)
    i. Classification
    ii. Life cycle: trophozoite, cysts;

    eggs→larva→adult
    iii. Definitive hosts and intermediate hosts
    iv. Protozoa: amebas, sporozoans, flagellates, cilates
    v. Helminthes: Platyhelminthes and Nemathelminthes
      a. Platyhelminthes have two classes: Cestodes (tapeworms) and Trematoda (flukes)
  b) Intestinal and urogenital protozoa (1hr)
    i. Intestinal protozoa
      a. Entamoeba
      b. Giardia
      c. Cryptosporidium
    ii. Urogenital Protozoa
      a. Trichomonas
  c) Blood and tissue protozoa (1hr)
    i. Sporozoans
      a. Plasmodium (malaria)-P. falciparum, P. vivax, P. malariae, P. ovale
    ii. Toxoplasma
  d) Flagellates (1/2hr)
    i. Trypanosoma
    ii. Leishmania
  e) Cestodes (tapeworm) (1/2hr)
    i. Distinguishing features
      a. Anatomy
      b. Reproduction and intermediate hosts
    ii. Diphyllbothrium latum
    iii. Echinococcus granulosus
  f) Nematodes (1/2hr)
  g) Trematodes (1/2hr)

Training Exercises	• Visit microbiology labs integrated with theory classes. • Videos should be used for individual or group study because it can be rewound or forwarded for better understanding of concepts. • Prepare lecture and hand-outs for the relevant topics to be presented. • The student is encouraged to research on topic prior to the lesson so that the lesson reinforces already learnt material or informative discussions can be held with the class or trainer. • Case studies may be done at the clinics to enhance contact with actual patients and presented in class to enhance communication and problem solving skills. • Models allow the student to touch the material and practice handling procedures prior to the actual human contact. • Computer-based learning materials like videos can be stored for continuous revision and conceptualisation of the topic.
Measurement based on Module Objectives	The trainer may choose to use any or all of the following: • Research reports • Assignments • Small group / whole group presentations • Written tests • Journals: Encourage the student to keep a weekly or monthly journal or course-based journal to enable him/her correlate all concepts which build into medicine. • Portfolios: Encourage the student to store all experiences (both successes and failures and make a continuous reflection on the topic). • Summative assessments will be done at the end of the topic or module or semester.
Relevance to Course to other modules or Practice	To offer the student a general overview of the biomedical sciences along with the professional competency development (PCD) and social and Population Health components. Complemented by longitudinal courses of professional competency development (PCD): history of medicine (International and national) and traditional medicine in Context country. Social and population health (SPH) courses: Introduction to determinants of health and health care advocacy.
Student Hand-outs	• Provide hand-outs based on lecture notes, Trainer's research, audio-visual materials • Provide hand-outs compiled from collaborative and group work presentations • Individual research reports may also be compiled for class references. • Case presentation reports may also be compiled for class references.

Audio-Visual Materials / Special Equipment / Resources Required	You may choose to use any or all of the following: • Multimedia equipment including: computer, LCD projector, Video, VCDs, DVDs, CD- ROMs • White board with white board marker or Blackboard with chalk • Models • Hospital wards / labs • Classroom or lab • Paper and hand-outs
Reference Materials	1. W.E. Levinson *Review of Medical Microbiology, 10th Ed.* (2008); Lange McGraw-Hill. ISB0071496023/ISB-13 978-0071496209 2. G.F. Brooks, J.S. Butel, K.C. Carroll, and S. A. Morse Jawetz, Melnick, and Adelberg's Medical Microbiology, 24th Edition; (2007); Appleton and Lange; ISB 0071287353/ISB-13 978-0071287357 3. L. M. de la Maza, et al. Color Atlas of Diagnostic Microbiology, Second Edition (2004); ASM Press;ISBN 1555812066 4. K. J. Ryan, Ed. Sherris Medical Microbiology, 4th Ed. (2003); Appleton & Lange; ISBN 0838585299 5. P.R. Murray et al. Medical Microbiology, 6th Ed., (2008); Moseby-Elsevier ISBN 0323054706/ISB-13 978-0323054706 6. eBook: RWJMS Microbiology and Immunology 7. P. H. Gilligan, M. L. Smiley, and D. S. Shapiro, Cases in Medical Microbiology and Infectious Diseases, 3rd Ed.(2003); ASM Press 8. Jawetz, Melnick and Adelberg's Medical Microbiology

Immunology

Course / Subject: Immunology
Course / Subject Time Distribution: Lectures - 8 Hours PBL - 4 Hours IL - 2 Hours WGS - 2 Hours

Course Objectives	By the end of this course the student is expected: 1. To describe the different forms of immune response and enumerate types of immunities. 2. To explain antigen-antibody reactions and describe the complement system. 3. To describe the pathogenesis of hypersensitivity reactions, autoimmune diseases and Immune deficiency states.

Course Content	1. Specific immune response,
	2. Nonspecific immune response,
	3. Responses,
	4. The cellular immune responses,
	5. The complement system,
	6. The different forms of immune response and
	7. Enumerate types of immunization,
	8. Antigen-antibody reactions and
	9. The pathogenesis of Hypersensitivity reactions,
	10. Autoimmune diseases and
	11. Immune deficiency states.
	12. Introduction to Immunology
	   1. Overview of the Immune system and the basis of immunity
	     a) Definitions
	       i. Antigen
	       ii. Immun responce
	       iii. Innet (natural) Immunity
	       iv. Aquired Immunity
	       v. The immun memory
	     b) Embryology: origin of immunologic agents including stem cells
	     c) Cells tissue and organs of the immun systems
	       i. Lymphositts
	       ii. Macrophages
	       iii. Dendritic cells
	       iv. Lymphoid tissue and Organs
	     d) Anatomy: sites of function of immunologic cells
	       i. RES
	       ii. Lymph nodes
	       iii. blood

e) Histology: microscopic appearance and function of immunologic agents (neutrophils, lymphocytes, macrophages, eosinophils, basophils, mast cells)
f) Antibodies and antigens
g) Immune system: Components of the immune system,
   i. Humoral immunity
   ii. Cellular immunity
h) Function: Types of immune system functions
   i. Barriers to entry
   ii. Innate immunity-exists prior to exposure; nonspecific; does not improve after exposure
   iii. Adaptive (Acquired) immunity-does not exist prior to exposure; specific; improves after exposre
      – Cell-mediated immunity
      – Antibody-mediated (humoral) immunity
      – T lymphocytes
      – B lymphocytes
      – Antibodies
         o Neutralize toxins and viruses
         o Opsonize bacteria
      – Functions of lymphocytes and mechanism of achieve
         o Diversity
         o Memory
         o Specificity
         o Inflammatory response
         o Phagocytes
      – Specificity
         o Recognition
         o Activation
         o response
i) Cell-mediated immunity
   i. Antigen (epitopes)
   ii. Class II Major Histocompatibility Complex (MHC)
   iii. Helper T lymphocytes
   iv. Cytotoxic T lypphocytes
   v. Class I Major Histocompatibility Complex (MHC)
   vi. Interleukins
j) Antibody-mediated Immunity
   i. Macrophages
   ii. Helper t cells
   iii. B cells
   iv. IL-2 (T-cell growth factor), IL-4 (B-cell growth factor), IK-5 (B-cell differentiation factor)

	2. Innate(Natural) Immunity
	  a) Killing invading microbes
	  b) Activating adaptive immune processes
	  c) Pathogen associated molecular patterns (PAMP) including toll-like receptors
	  d) Acute phase response
	  e) Defensins
	3. Acquired Immunity Components
	  a) Long term memory cells for adaptive immunity
	  b) Antigen presenting cells (Dendritic cells, macrophages, B cells)
	  c) Major histocompatibility complex I & II
	  d) Complement
	  e) Antigen presenting cells
	  f) lymphocytes
	  g) Antibodies
	4. Adaptive and passive immunity
	  a) Passive immunity: transferring preformed antibodies from another host to provide resistance; fast onset but temporary
	  b) Acquired immunity: acquired after contact with foreign antigen; long term but slow onset
	5. Clinical sequellae
	  a) Hypersensitivity
	    i. Type I: Immediate hypersensitivity (anaphylaxis)
	    ii. Type II: Cytotoxic hypersensitive
	    iii. Type III: Immune Complex Hypersensitivity
	    iv. Type IV: Delayed (cell-mediated) hypersensitivity
	  b) Autoimmune diseases
	  c) immunodeficiencies

Training Exercises	• Prepare lecture and hand-outs for the topics to be presented. • The student is encouraged to research on topic prior to the lesson so that the lesson reinforces already learnt material or informative discussions can be held with the class or trainer • Computer-based learning materials like videos may be stored for continuous revision and conceptualisation.
Measurement based on Module Objectives	You may choose to use any or all the following: • Research reports • Assignments • Small group / whole group presentations • Written tests • Journals: Encourage the student to keep a weekly or monthly journal or course-based journal to enable him/her correlate all concepts which build into medicine.

	• Portfolios: Encourage the student to store all experiences (both successes and failures and make a continuous reflection on the topic). • Summative assessments will be done at the end of the topic or module or semester.
Relevance to Course to other modules or Practice	• To offer the student a general overview of the biomedical sciences along with the professional competency development (PCD) and social and Population Health components. • Complemented by longitudinal courses of professional competency development (PCD): history of medicine (International and national) and traditional medicine in Context country. Social and population health (SPH) courses: Introduction to determinants of health and health care advocacy.
Student Hand-outs	• Provide hand-outs based on lecture notes, your research, audio-visual materials • Provide hand-outs compiled from collaborative and group work presentations • Individual research reports may also be compiled for class references. • Case presentation reports may also be compiled for class references.
Audio-Visual Materials / Special Equipment / Resources Required	You may choose to use any or all of the following: • Multimedia equipment including: computer, LCD projector, Video, VCDs, DVDs, CD- ROMs • White board with white board marker or available resource • Models • Classroom / Labs • Hospital wards / Labs • Paper and hand-outs
Reference Materials	1. Mims, Dockrell, Goering, Roitt; *Mims et al. Medical Microbiology*, 3rd Ed 2004, Elsevier

Pharmacology

Course / Subject: Pharmacology
Course / Subject Time Distribution: Lectures - 20 Hours PBL - 4 Hours IL - 7 Hours WGS - 10 Hours

Course Objectives	By the end of this course the student is expected: 1. To describe and internalize the scope of pharmacology 2. To define pharmacology and discuss on the different sources of drugs 3. To discuss on the different sources of drugs, routes of drug administration, pharmacokinetics, dosage and dosage regime, pharmacodynamics, factors modifying drug effects, drug interactions, adverse drug reactions, and new drug development.

Course Content	1. Different sources of drugs
	2. Routes of drug administration
	3. Pharmacokinetics
	4. Dosage and dosage regime
	5. Pharmacodynamics
	6. Factors modifying drug effects
	7. Drug interactions
	8. Adverse drug reactions
	a) Basic Principles In pharmacology
	  1. Introduction (total 3 hours)
	    – Definitions and history: pharmacology (5 min)
	    – Pharmacology & genetics(7 min)
	    – The nature of drugs (7 min)
	  2. The physical nature of drugs(7 min)
	  3. Drug size(7 min)
	  4. Drug reactivity and drug-receptor bonds(7 min)
	  5. Drug shape(7 min)
	  6. Rational drug design (7 min)
	  7. Receptor nomenclature(7 min)
	  8. Drug-body interactions(10 min)
	  9. Pharmacodynamic principles (7 min)
	  10. Duration of drug action (7 min)
	  11. Receptors and inert binding sites(7 min)
	  12. Pharmacokinetic principles(7 min)
	  13. Permeation(5 min)
	  14. Aqueous diffusion(5 min)
	  15. Lipid diffusion(5 min)
	  16. Special carriers(5 min)
	  17. Endocytosis and exocytosis(5min)
	  18. Drug groups(5 min)

b) Drug receptors & pharmacodynamics

1. Drug receptors & pharmacodynamics: introduction
2. Macromolecular nature of drug receptors
3. Relation between drug concentration & response
4. Concentration-effect curves & receptor binding of agonists
5. Receptor-effector coupling & spare receptors
6. Competitive & irreversible antagonists
7. Partial agonists
8. Other mechanisms of drug antagonism
9. Cytokine receptors
10. Ligand-gated channels
11. G proteins & second messengers
12. Receptor regulation
13. Well-established second messengers
    a. Cyclic adenosine monophosphate (cAMP)
    b. Calcium and phosphoinositides
    c. Cyclic guanosine monophosphate (cGMP)
    d. Interplay among signaling mechanisms
    e. Phosphorylation: a common theme
    f. Receptor classes & drug development
    g. Relation between drug dose & clinical response
14. Dose & response in patients
    a. Graded dose-response relations
    b. Potency
    c. Maximal efficacy
    d. Shape of dose-response curves
    e. Quantal dose-effect curves
    f. Variation in drug responsiveness
    g. Alteration in concentration of drug that reaches the receptor
    h. Variation in concentration of an endogenous receptor ligand
    i. Alterations in number or function of receptors
    j. Changes in components of response distal to the receptor
15. Clinical selectivity:
    a. Beneficial versus toxic effects of drugs
    b. Beneficial and toxic effects mediated by the same receptor-effector mechanism
    c. Beneficial and toxic effects mediated by identical receptors but in different tissues or by different effector pathways
    d. Beneficial and toxic effects mediated by different types of receptors

c) **Pharmacokinetics & pharmacodynamics:**
1. Rational dosing & the time course of drug action: introduction
2. Pharmacokinetics
3. Volume of distribution
4. Capacity-limited elimination
5. Flow-dependent elimination
6. Half-life
7. Drug accumulation
8. Bioavailability
9. Extent of absorption
10. First-pass elimination
11. Rate of absorption
12. Extraction ratio & the first-pass effect
13. Alternative routes of administration & the first-pass effect
14. The time course of drug effect
15. Immediate effects
16. Delayed effects
17. Cumulative effects
18. The target concentration approach to designing a rational dosage regimen
19. Maintenance dose
20. Loading dose
21. Therapeutic drug monitoring: relating pharmacokinetics & pharmacodynamics
22. The target concentration strategy
23. Pharmacokinetic variables
    a. Absorption
    b. Clearance
    c. Volume of distribution
    d. Half-life
    e. Pharmacodynamic variables
24. Pharmacodynamic variables
    a. Maximum effect
    b. Sensitivity
25. Interpretation of drug concentration measurements
    a. Clearance
    b. Plasma protein binding: is it important?
    c. Dosing history
    d. Timing of samples for concentration measurement
26. Initial predictions of volume of distribution & clearance
    a. Volume of distribution
    b. Clearance
    c. Revising individual estimates of volume of distribution & clearance

d) Drug biotransformation
  1. Drug biotransformation: introduction
  2. Why is drug biotransformation necessary?
  3. Where do drug biotransformation occur?
  4. Microsomal mixed function oxidase system & phase i
  5. Reactionsenzyme
  6. Inductionhuman liver P450 enzymes
  7. Drug biotransformation: introduction why is drug biotransformation necessary?
  8. Where do drug biotransformations occur?
  9. Microsomal mixed function oxidase system & phase i
  10. Reactions
  11. Enzyme induction
  12. Enzyme inhibition
  13. Human liver P450 enzymes
  14. Phase ii reactions
  15. Metabolism of drugs to toxic products
  16. Clinical relevance of drug metabolism
      a) Individual differences
      b) Genetic factors
      c) Diet & environmental factors
      d) Age & sex
      e) Drug-drug interactions during metabolism
      f) Diseases affecting drug metabolism
      g) Interactions between drugs & endogenous compounds
  17. Diseases affecting drug metabolism
e) Basic & clinical evaluation of new drugs
  1. Basic & clinical evaluation of new drugs: introduction
  2. Drug discovery
  3. Drug screening
  4. Preclinical safety & toxicity testing
  5. Evaluation in humans
  6. Confounding factors in clinical trials
  7. The variable natural history of most diseases
  8. The presence of other diseases and risk factors
  9. Subject and observer bias
  10. The presence of other diseases and risk factors
  11. Subject and observer bias
  12. The food & drug administration
  13. Clinical trials: The IND & NDA
  14. Orphan drugs
  15. Adverse reactions to drugs
  16. Evaluating a clinical drug study
  17. Research, development, & marketing

Training Exercises	• Integrated labs to complement theory work • Prepare lecture and hand-outs for the relevant topics to be presented. • The student is encouraged to research on topic prior to the lesson so that the lesson reinforces already learnt material or informative discussions can be held with the class or trainer • Case studies may be done at the clinics to enhance contact with actual patients and presented in class to enhance communication and problem solving skills. • Computer-based learning materials like videos can be stored for continuous revision and conceptualisation of the topic.
Measurement based on Module Objectives	You may choose to use any or all of the following: • Research reports • Assignments • Small group / whole group presentations • Written tests • Journals: Encourage the student to keep a weekly or monthly journal or course-based journal to enable him/her correlate all concepts which build into medicine. • Portfolios: Encourage the student to store all experiences (both successes and failures and make a continuous reflection on the topic). • Summative assessments will be done at the end of the topic or module or semester.
Relevance to Course to other modules or Practice	• To offer the student a general overview of the biomedical sciences along with the professional competency development (PCD) and social and Population Health components. • Complemented by longitudinal courses of professional competency development (PCD): history of medicine (International and national) and traditional medicine in Context country. Social and population health (SPH) courses: Introduction to determinants of health and health care advocacy.
Student Hand-outs	• Provide hand-outs based on lecture notes, Trainer's research, audio-visual materials • Provide hand-outs compiled from collaborative and group work presentations • Individual research reports may also be compiled for class references. • Case presentation reports may also be compiled for class references.

Audio-Visual Materials / Special Equipment / Resources Required	You may choose to use any or all of the following: • Multimedia equipment including: computer, LCD projector, Video, VCDs, DVDs, CD- ROMs • White board with white board marker or available resource • Models, Classroom/ Labs, Paper and Hand-outs
Reference Materials	1. **Goodman & Gilman's The Pharmacological Basis of Therapeutics. 11th Edition,** Laurence Brunton, John Lazo, Keith Parker, Eds., McGraw Hill, New York, 2006. 2. Basic and Clinical Pharmacology, 11th Ed., Bertram G. Katzung, Susan B. Masters, Anthony J. Trevor, 2009, McGraw-Hill (Lange Series) ISBN13:9780071604055 3. Wecker, L., G. Dunaway, and C. Faingold. *Human Pharmacology: Molecular to Clinical.* 5th edition, 2009. Elsevier. 4. Page, C. et al. *Integrated Pharmacology.* 3rd edition, 2006. Mosby-Yearbook. $84. Good for ***problem-based curriculum***. Organized by disease rather than drug class. 5. Katzung and Trevor's Pharmacology, Examination and Board Review, Eight Edition Edited by Anthony J. Trevor, Bertram G. Katzung, Susan Masters a Lange Medical Book published by McGraw Hill 2008 6. Applied Therapeutics: The Clinical Use of Drugs 7. Principles of pharmacologic pathologic bases of drug therapy 8. Craig, C. R., and R. E. Stitzel, eds. *Modern Pharmacology with Clinical Applications.* 6th edition, 2004. Lippincott, Williams & Wilkins. $65. 9. Golan, D. et al. *Principles of Pharmacology: The Pathophysiologic Basis of Drug Therapy.* 2nd edition, 2008. Lippincott Williams & Wilkins.

Section IB

Integrated Biomedical
Laboratory Practice

Integrated Laboratory Sessions in Preclinical Courses

Planning for Demonstrations

You may use the following steps to prepare for demonstration lessons or laboratory sessions.

1. Develop demonstrations and role plays by breaking down the task into sequential steps (Task Analysis). You can do this for all procedures.
2. Once the steps are outlined, you must demonstrate the steps to the student either in the lab or in the clinic as she/he observes.
3. Allow the student to practice the steps.
4. Ask the student to demonstrate the procedure.
5. Give feedback at the end to correct inconsistencies or missing links
6. Ask the student to practice again with the corrections
7. Each and every student must practice the skill.

Objectives

At the end of the practical sessions, the student will be able to:

1. Identify the normal disposition, inter-relationships, gross anatomy of the skeleton and axis's of movement of the various structures
2. Describe the differnt types of joints
3. Identify different kinds of tissues and organs
4. Describe the standard procedures in the preparation of histological specimen
5. Identify different types of commonly used histological stains
6. Identify ovum and sperm cell and early phase of embryogenesis

Content

Combination of all outlined contents of Anatomy, Histology and Embryology

Learning Activities and Resources
- Learning guide and checklist
- Prepared slides different tissues
- Video microscope or microscope
- LCD projector or slide projector
- Computer

Gross Anatomy

Objectives

At the end of this practical session, the student will be able to:
1. Differentiate descriptive terms and different body movements in anatomy including terms of position and relation
2. To demonstrate an understanding of the nature and organization of the major, grossly visible structural components of the dissected human body

Content
- Demonstration of terms in anatomy including terms of position and relation
- The different body movements:
  - o Axes of movement (longitudinal, sagittal, transverse or horizontal)
  - o movements-lateral and medial rotation, flexion and extension, abduction and adduction, circumduction,
  - o Human skeleton structure and joints

Learning Activities
- Demonstration using anatomical models
- Computer-assisted learning
- Dissection of cadaver
- Skeleton audit

Learning resources
- Learning guide and checklist
- Anatomical models
- Cadaver
- Human skeleton
- CD-ROM
- Computer

Formative assessment
- You may use a computer-assisted test
- You may design and give a quiz at the end of session.

Histology

Objectives

At the end of this practical session, the student will be able to:
1. Illustrate the structure and basic parts (nucleus and cytoplasm) of a cell.
2. Explain the different types of tissues & glands.
3. Describe the standard procedures in the preparation of histological specimen
4. Demonstrate an understanding of the different types of commonly used histological stains.

Content
1. Use of Microscopy
2. Standard procedures in the preparation of histological specimen
3. Different types of commonly used histological stains
4. The cell
5. The different types of Epithelial cells and tissues
6. The different types of Connective Tissue & supportive tissue

Learning Activities
- Microscopy
- Demonstration commonly used stains in histology
- Demonstration and practice on histological specimen
- Slide show of the tissues

Learning resources
- Learning guide and checklist
- Prepared slides different tissues
- Video microscope or microscope
- LCD projector or slide projector
- Computer

Formative assessment
- **Computer-assisted test** (Identifying macroscopic and microscopic structures of the embryonic development)
- Design a quiz at the end of session.

Embryology

Objectives

At the end of this practical session, the student will be able to:
1. Describe basic human embryologic development
2. Describe intrauterine developmental anatomy of the human embryo including the common embryonic anomalies from conception to organogenesis.

Content
1. Sperm and ova
2. Morula blastula spermatogenesis
3. The different stages in the development of the embryo
4. Common embryonic anomalies from conception to organogenesis

Learning Activities
- Demonstration of anatomical charts and models
- Video show
- Slide show
- Computer-assisted learning

Learning Resources
- Learning guide and checklist
- Anatomical charts and models of different stages of embryo development
- Prepared slides of serial section of the embryo at different stages
- CD-ROM of embryonic development
- Video microscope or microscope
- LCD projector or slide projector
- Computer.

Formative assessment
- Computer-assisted test (Identifying macroscopic and microscopic structures of the embryonic development)
- Quiz at the end of session.

Physiology

Objectives
At the end of this practical session, the student will be able to:
1. Illustrate the structure and basic parts (nucleus and cytoplasm) of a cell Illustrate the structure and function of cell membrane including:
2. Differentiate components of plasma membrane, membrane transport of molecules, diffusion, active transport, cell signalling, membrane potential, action potential

Content
1. Cells as the living units of the body
2. Extracellular Fluid-The "Internal Environment"
3. "Homeostatic" Mechanisms of the Major Functional Systems
4. DNA synthesis
5. RNA synthesis

6. Membrane physiology and signalling
7. Special Characteristics of Signal Transmission in Nerve Trunks
8. Function and structure of the skeletal muscle

Learning Activities
- Illustration s through DVD/ VCD
- Website for learning
- Observe activities of the skeletal muscle on a lab animal (such as frog).

Learning Resources
- Learning guide and checklist
- Lab animal such as frog
- Timer

Formative Assessment
- Quiz or Computer-assisted test at the end of the session.

Biochemistry

Objectives
By the end of the practical session the student will be able to:
1. Observe determination of lipid profile and enzymes in a hospital lab or integrated basic science lab
2. Demonstrate Nucleic acids: DNA and RNA structure and replication on computer simulation,
3. Nutrition: Energy calculations

Content
- DNA Transcription
- Post-transcriptional processing
- Translation of genetic code
- Regulation of gene expression and protein synthesis inhibitors of protein synthesis
- DNA repair mechanisms
- Serum lipids

- Nutrient effects in weight management and fitness (fat and glycogen metabolism)
- BMI

Learning Activities
- Observe laboratory tests to determine serum lipids in hospital or integrated basic sciences lab
- Computer simulation exercise of DNA structure

Learning Resources
- Learning guide and checklist
- Blood chemistry analyser
- Reagents
- Blood sample

Pathology

Objective
1. Identify gross and microscopic alteration of tissues and organs of the CVS in disease processes and conditions

Content
1. Cell injury, adaptation and death
2. General pathology of infectious diseases
3. Acute and chronic inflammation
4. Tissue repair: cell regeneration and fibrosis
5. Hemodynamic disorders, thrombosis, and shock
6. Neoplasia

Learning Activities
- Observation of pathological specimens and slides in lab and electronic museum
- Attend post-mortem examinations

Learning Resources
- Learning guide and checklist
- Pathology specimens
- Pathology slides
- Electronic museum of pathological lesions
- Video microscope or microscope
- LCD projector and computer
- Slide projector

Microbiology and Parasitology

Objectives
At the end of the practical session the student should be able to:
1. Identify steps in collecting samples for gram staining and culture
2. Identify the culture media used to grow common bacteria involved in infections
3. Classify steps and sequence of gram staining and culture
4. Differentiate gram positive and gram negative bacteria
5. Demonstrate an understanding of the concepts on growth of bacteria in a culture media

Content
1. Gram staining
2. Culture media (bacteria)

Learning activities
- Microscopy and micrometry
- Direct demonstration of bacteria by staining
- Motility tests and biochemical tests for bacterial identification
- Laboratory diagnosis of viral infections
- Laboratory diagnosis of fungal infections
- Sterilization and disinfection
- Participate in performing gram staining technique
- Observe preparation of bacteriological culture media
- Participate in performing laboratory diagnosis of selected common bacteria.

Learning Resources
- Learning guide and checklist
- Reagents and slides for gram stain
- Ingredients for culture media
- Microscope
- Test samples (throat swab and blood)

Pharmacology

Objective

By the end of the pharmacology practical, the student will be able to:
1. Illustrate pharmacological effects of basic drugs on the heart and blood vessels using computer simulation

Content
1. Different sources of drugs
2. Routes of drug administration
3. Pharmacokinetics
4. Dosage and dosage regime
5. Pharmacodynamics
6. Factors modifying drug effects
7. Drug interactions
8. Adverse drug reactions

Learning Activities
- Demonstration and practice on computer-aided simulation
- Lab processes and procedures

Learning Resources
- Learning guide and checklist
- Computers
- Pharmacology simulation program

Section II

Professional Competency
Development (PCD)

PCD Course Description and Course Design

Course overview

The PCD component of the medical curriculum intends to develop a student who not only has clinical skills but also generic skills in communication, ethics and professionalism. This course intends to give an understanding of current codes of conducts in professionalism and the role recognition that is required of medics.

Design

Several themes will be covered that have been divided in the pre-clerkship and clerkship periods. The component is offered longitudinally alongside biomedical and social and population health courses offered during year 1. The course should be offered half (1/2) a day per week.

This section is divided into two parts:

1. Section **IIA** is a guide for professional competency coursework.
2. Section **IIB** is a guide for skills lab and hospital OPD practice.

Section IIA

Professional Competency
Development Courses

Duration: 40 Weeks (Years 1-4)

Introduction to Learning Methods

Course / Subject: Introduction to Learning Methods	
Course / Subject Time Distribution: Lectures - 6 Hours SGS - 2 Hours WGS - 2 Hours CRL - 2 Hours	
Course Objectives	By the end of this course, the student will be able to: 1. Describe the components of the medical curriculum and take active responsibility for his/her learning. 2. Recognize the gross structure and design of the medical curriculum 3. Demonstrate understanding of principles underlying the curriculum design 4. Describe the minimum essential competencies required of a medic 5. Demonstrate understanding of the teaching-learning methods to be used in the curriculum with focus on student-driven methods 6. Describe the assessment methods including grading and promotion criteria to be used in the curriculum with focus on student-driven methods.
Course Content	1. Overview of structure and design of the medical curriculum 2. Principles and strategies underpinning the medical curriculum 3. Core competencies of the context country's medical doctor 4. Suggested teaching-learning methods with focus on student-driven methods in the medical curriculum 5. Suggested student assessment methods (including grading and promotion criteria) with focus on student driven methods.
Training Exercises	• Small group and large group discussion: browse through the curriculum document • In small group discussion (SGD): question and answer with clarifications • Interactive presentation / lecture: explain the principles and strategies of the curriculum and addresses students' questions. • SGS and WGS: student review core competencies expected of a medical doctor. Each small group focuses on one broad domain. They will use creative methods like brief role play or story to demonstrate what that domain represents. • Interactive presentation: explain the teaching/learning methods with focus on new and student-driven approaches. • In small groups: student review sample tools that exemplify the teaching-learning methods such as PRRE and reflective portfolio • Give demonstrations (or shows video) of a PBL session e.g. in small groups student should conduct role plays of a PBL session

	• Interactive presentation: explanation of the assessment methods with focus on new and student-driven approaches, in small groups student review sample assessment tools and templates • Student practice completing student-driven assessment tools such as reflective portfolio and 360 degree evaluation using the sessions and group activities as a point of focus • Facilitate discussion in the plenary answering remaining questions and discussing results of the activities
Measurement based on Module Objectives	• You may assess the student based on assignments or presentations from SGDs or role plays.
Relevance to Course to other modules or Practice	This course introduces the medical student to the curriculum and helps the student to internalise the expected competencies of context country's medical doctor. The student will have an opportunity to discuss all parts of the curriculum.
Student Hand-outs	You may develop hand-outs highlighting the key points of the curriculum including teaching and learning methods and activities, expected competencies, assessment methods, time lines and deadlines
Audio-Visual Materials / Special Equipment / Resources Required	You may choose to use any or all of the following: • Multimedia equipment including: computer, LCD projector, Video, VCDs, DVDs, CD- ROMs • White board with white board marker or available resource • Models / standardised patients.
Reference Materials	The curriculum, assessment templates and relevant supportive websites should be provided for the student.

Study Skills

Course / Subject: Study Skills	
Course / Subject Time Distribution: Lecture / WGS - 3 Hours	
Course Design/ Description	This course will assist the student to deal with the challenges of studying effectively in medical school. It introduces the student to effective study techniques with the aim of guiding the student towards mastery of material and not just memorization. It also seeks to build confidence in critical thinking and applying knowledge effectively. The ability to study effectively and efficiently is important for the student as the basis for which they learn how to think critically during clerkship years. The course will help the student to internalise the concepts of student oriented and competency based teaching and learning.
Course Objectives	By the end of this course the student will be able to: 1. Develop effective studying skills 2. Distinguish areas of study that require memorization alone from those both requiring both memorization 3. Identify several models of studying and be able to choose which style fits them.

Course Content	• Clarify some reasons why becoming a good doctor involves intentional hard work:
	   o Evolving understanding of science and medicine
	   o Importance of time management
	   o Large volume of data to recall
	   o Need to sort through lots of material
	 • Demonstrate range of materials that need to be internalized
	   o Charts
	   o Algorithms
	   o Diagrams
	   o Visual images
	   o Detailed anatomic structure
	   o Mechanisms
	   o Exceptions to rules
	 • Reinforce that
	   o Mastery and memorization are related but different
	   o A great student, good student, and poor student are separated only by effectiveness of studying
	   o Cramming material last second is not effective nor sustainable
	 • Review individual topics that feature
	   o Anatomy: function, charts to memorize, rules and exception
	   o sHistology: function, physiology, and correlate to structures visualized on slide

- o Physiology: structures, sequence of mechanism and normal variations
- o Microbiology: agent, mechanism of entry, life cycle, sites of biologic activity within host and response elicited, host presentation, and treatment
- o Pharmacology: drug, mechanism of action, target, duration of activity, Class side effect, factors that affect pharmacokinetics
- o Pathophysiology: normal physiology, basis for pathology, mechanism of disease, microscopic/macroscopic/clinical presentation
- Mistakes (discourage):
  - o Cramming the day before the test
  - o Learning new material the day before the test
  - o Only reading and re-reading the material-take your own note
- Review approaches to topics
  - o Surveying-prior to lecture, skimming material to be studied-charts, diagrams, headings of sections and paragraphs; organize material chronologically, structurally, in stages, or in importance
  - o Concept mapping technique-highlighting and attaching questions to actively learn the material
  - o Sketching pieces of material to reinforce interconnection of material-diagrams, charts, pictures,
  - o Group study or Peer teaching-teaching requires the student to organize the material and present it in a way that is conceptually simple enough for his peers to understand but also applies the details to their understanding
- s• Goals:
  - o Review all material at least 5 times
  - o Review the material 3 times within the first 24 hours, the time period scientifically shown to be most critical for learning
  - o Review the material at least 2 more times by the test date (the weekend of the material and a general review several days before the test)
- Integrating all of these techniques
  - o Preview: look at the lecture materials beforehand if possible and if not possible then the lecture objectives. Actively review it by either:
    - ▪ Summarize it in 5-10 sentences (Why: gives you a roadmap of the lecture
    - ▪ Write down 5-10 questions that the lecture should answer

	○ Lecture: Encourage the student to ensure that the lecture answers his/her questions or addresses all summary. If not, encouarage the student to always approach the professor for clarifications. If still not clear, consult the textbook and to keep all avenues for learning open. ○ Post lecture: ▪ Briefly summarize the lecture and book into your own words (not copying what was said or written) ▪ Diagram what was said; goal-5 diagrams per lecture ▪ Make sure you understand everything ○ Review: key: How to add sentences to your notes linking concept to something else ▪ #1: the day after the lecture-learning requires consolidation of details which requires repeated exposures. No more than 10-15min per subject per day.
	▪ #2: skim lecture for main points; add to it ▪ #3: weekend review: master review of all material. ▪ #4: read through your own notes • Introduce questions as important learning devices: ○ Questions reinforce what you know ○ The answers to questions may cover material you do not know ○ Questions may address areas in which you are weak and need improvement ○ Questions address practical aspects of the material
Training Exercises	You may use the following: • Interactive lectures • Assignments • Individual study projects • Whole group discussion and presentations • Journals: Encourage the student to keep a weekly or monthly journal or course-based journal to enable him/her correlate all concepts which build into medicine. • Portfolios: Encourage the student to store all experiences (both successes and failures and make a continuous reflection on the topic).
Measurement based on Module Objectives	Assessment may not be required but the student is encouraged to keep journals and portfolios concerning his/her study progress.
Relevance to Course to other modules or Practice	This course provides the medical student with effective study skills which will help him/her to acquire the expected competencies. These study skills will be carried over throughout the career into lifelong learning.

Student Hand-outs	• Hand-outs should be provided detailing the models of effective study skills • Provide hand-outs based on lecture notes, your research, audio-visual materials • Provide hand-outs compiled from collaborative and group work presentations • Individual research reports may also be compiled for class references. • You may also compile case presentation reports for class references.
Audio-Visual Materials / Special Equipment / Resources Required	You may choose to use any or all of the following: • Multimedia equipment including: computer, LCD projector, Video, VCDs, DVDs, CD- ROMs • White board with white board marker or available resource
Reference Materials	Provide the student with Bibliographies, Websites, Library, E resources and relevant references.

History of Medicine in the World and the context country

Course / Subject: History of Medicine in the world and the context country	
Course / Subject Time Distribution: Lectures - 5 Hours WGS - 2 Hours	
Course Description	With the existing study of the history of medicine this course will reinforce the professional values, the scientific understanding and the social commitment of the future new graduate. Medicine in context country will also be taught.
Course Objectives	As a result of studying in this short course, the student will be able to: 1. Relate historic attitudes and the values of the doctor to those which were developed in the Hippocratic School. Therefore the course will study Hippocrates and his times and the values of the ancients. 2. Describe how the Renaissance brought new discipline to the practice of medicine and introduced new studies and how, for example, Leonardo de Vinci and William Harvey experimented and how their approach grew during the Enlightenment in Europe. Therefore the student will make a period study of major figures in medicine in the late Middle Ages and the Enlightenment. 3. Describe the advance of public health during the nineteenth century and the major advances which enable medicine of the 21ST century to be practised. Therefore the student will be able to describe, with reference to major public health issues in Context country and to current clinical practice, how changes have been based on scientific advance and evidence. 4. Describe one major communicable disease and how its control and treatment have developed and been influenced by scientific, social and political events in Africa or in Context country.
Course Content	1. Hippocrates and his times and the values of the ancients, major figures in medicine in the late middle Ages and the Enlightenment, 2. Reference to major public health issues in context country and to current clinical practice, how changes have been based on scientific advance and evidence. 3. History of major communicable disease and how its control and treatment have developed and been influenced by scientific, social and political events in context country (Malaria, TB, HIV/AID, Leprosy)
Training Exercises	• Lectures: Prepare lectures and hand-outs • Self-directed learning (SDL): Advice the student to research on the topics prior to the lesson so that the lesson reinforces or informative discussions can be held with the class or trainer • E-Learning on the net and computer-based learning materials

Measurement based on Module Objectives	You may use any or all of the following: • Project work • Quizzes • Research reports • Assignments • WGS/ Class / group presentations • Written tests • Journals: Encourage the student to keep a weekly or monthly journal or course-based journal to enable him/her correlate all concepts which build into medicine. • Portfolios: Encourage the student to store all experiences (both successes and failures and make a continuous reflection on the topic). • Summative assessments will be done at the end of the topic or module or semester.
Relevance to Course to other modules or Practice	Reinforce the professional values, the scientific understanding and the social commitment of the future.
Student Hand-outs	• Provide hand-outs based on lecture notes, your research, audio-visual materials • Provide hand-outs compiled from collaborative and group work presentations • Individual research reports may also be compiled for class references. • You may also compile case presentation reports for class references.
Audio-Visual Materials / Special Equipment / Resources Required	• Multimedia equipment including: computer, LCD projector, Video, VCDs, DVDs, CD- ROMs • White board with white board marker or available resource • Paper and hand-outs
Reference Materials	Provide the student with Bibliographies, Websites, Library and E resources and relevant references.

Clinical Skills

Course / Subject: Clinical Skills	
Course / Subject Time Distribution: Lectures - 10 Hours IL - 18 Hours	
Course Description	To enable the student to apply their basic science concepts and critical thinking skills in clinical practice. It also aims to prepare student for the "real patient" contact they will encounter in their community practice, clinical clerkships intern ship and future practice. This will enable the student to acquire skill to collect data
	by interview physical examination and laboratory or radiological tests to make ethical and logical clinical decision making in the management of patients and to communicate effectively with patients and families and arrive at a satisfactory plan. The acquisition of professional skills will enable the student to acquire, synthesize, interpret and record clinical information. The fundamentals of these skills are to enable the student to communicate effectively with patients while recognizing their clinical problems in the context of behavioural and psychological needs. **The five major skills are:** • Physician –Patient communication skill • Clinical data collection • Hypothesis generation • Clinical decision making including ethical decisions • Inter- professional communication
Course Design	The clinical skills course is designed to develop and refine the clinical interview, physical examination and documentation skills of medical student. The student will be trained in the habits of proper communication, physical examination, critical analysis and documentation skills all of which are fundamental to the sound practice of medicine. Clinical skills will be offered in the Year I for 24 hrs in theory classes and for 3 hrs in every system for a total of 36 hrs based modules in skill lab and in clerkship integrated with the specific discipline.
Course Objectives	The learning objectives of the clinical skills course are for the student to demonstrate proficiency in the following skills and behaviours: 1. Obtaining a medical history. 2. Performing physical examinations. 3. Documenting and reporting the history and physical. 4. Providing effective patient education and counselling. 5. Professional conduct - engendering confidence in patients through appropriate dress and demeanour.

	6. Developing a good patient / physician relationship, including data gathering and interpersonal aspects.
	7. Understand the various causes of disease and the role that proper history taking and physical examination plays in uncovering pathology.
	8. Employ the scientific method when diagnosing conditions and when ascertaining the efficacy of traditional and non-traditional therapies.
	9. Understand the bio-psychosocial determinants of health and illness.
	10. Understand the principles of health promotion and disease prevention
	11. Demonstrate caring and respectful behaviour towards patients.
	12. Demonstrate consideration of patients' privacy, dignity and psychological needs.
	13. Demonstrate effective listening skills.
	14. Foster an ethical and therapeutic relationship with patients by cultivating mutual respect and trust.
	15. Demonstrate self-directed learning skills and progressive professional development.
Course Content	1. Medical history
	2. Physical examinations,
	3. Documenting and reporting the history and physical examination findings
	4. Effective patient education and counselling
	5. Professional conduct
	6. Development of good patient/physician relationship
	7. Including data gathering and interpersonal aspects
	8. Causes of disease and the role that proper history taking and physical examination plays in uncovering pathology
	9. Scientific methods of diagnosing conditions
	10. Efficacy of traditional and non-traditional therapies
	11. Bio-psychosocial determinants of health and illness
	12. Principles of health promotion and disease prevention,
	13. Empathy, respectful behaviour towards patients, patients' privacy, dignity and psychological needs, effective listening skills, ethical and therapeutic relationship with patients / mutual respect and trust
	14. Self-directed learning skills and progressive professional development skills

Training Exercises	You may use any of the following teaching and learning methods: • Lecture • Small group Sessions • Whole group session • Ambulatory clinical attachment • Skills lab and Integrated biomedical laboratory practical session • E-learning • Hospital Attachments • Mentorship • Self-directed Learning

Measurement based on Module Objectives	You may use any or all of the following:
	• DOCS (Direct Observation of Clinical Skills)
	• OSC/PE (Objective Structured Clinical / Practical Examination)
	• Oral exam (Viva)
	• Written exam (MCQ, Short Essay, Matching, True- False with reasoning)
	• Portfolios
	• Project work
	• Quizzes and written tests
	• Assignments
	• Whole group / small group presentations
	• Log books / Journals: Encourage the student to keep a weekly or monthly journal or course-based journal to enable him/her correlate all concepts which build into medicine.
	• Portfolios: Encourage the student to store all experiences (both successes and failures and make a continuous reflection on the topic).
	• **Summative assessment**
	  ○ Progressive (continuous) assessment (Quizzes, concept application exercise tutorial-based evaluation) 40%
	  ○ End of each system exam 60%
	• **Formative assessment**
	This will not contribute to the total grade of the student but provide continuous feedback to the student. You can conduct it in the form of providing feedback on completed assignments or student's professional behaviour

Relevance to Course to other modules or Practice	This course will enable the graduate to: • Manage patients in an effective, efficient and ethical manner including health promotion and disease prevention • Evaluate health problems and advise patients taking into account physical, psychological, social and cultural factors

Instruments and materials required for the student	• Stethoscope • Ophthalmoscope/Otoscope set • Sphygmomanometer (manual Blood Pressure kit): Standard Adult Cuff • (Required) Large and small adult and paediatric cuffs • Reflex hammer • Penlight • Tuning Fork (512 Hz frequency) • Near-vision Card (Eye Exam Overview • Details of Skill lab standards will be demonstrated in separate standards document.
Student Hand-outs	• Provide a student's guide • Conduct exercises that enable self-directed learning • Provide hand-outs based on lecture notes, your research, audio-visual materials • Provide hand-outs compiled from collaborative and group work presentations • Individual research reports may also be compiled for class references. • Case presentation reports may also be compiled for class references.
Audio-Visual Materials / Special Equipment	• Small Group session smaller rooms. • Skills lab • Flip Charts • IT centre with good internet connection • Clinical set up • Library Multimedia equipment including: computer, LCD projector, Video, VCDs, DVDs, CD- ROMs • White board with white board marker or available resource • Electric power • Classroom or Lab
Human Resources Required	• Clinicians • General Practitioner • Standardised patients • Other relevant Health Professionals (for Inter professional Pool)
Reference Materials	Provide the student with Bibliographies, Websites, Library and E resources and relevant references: 1. Edmariam Tsega *Guide to Physical Examination* 2. Health Assessment Online: **http://evolve.elsevier.com** 3. *Bates' Guide to Physical Examination* & History Taking (Book with CD-ROM) 4. Swartz, *Textbook of Physical Diagnosis,* 6th ed., 2009, Elsevier, ISBN-13: 9781416062035 5. Bickley, Lynn S. Bates' *Guide to Physical Examination and History Taking.* 10th Edition, Lippincott Williams and Wilkins C., 2009

Ethics and Legal Medicine

Course / Subject: Ethics and Legal Medicine	
Course / Subject Time Distribution: Lectures - 12 Hours SGS - 4 Hours	
Course Design/ Description	Ethics is one component of the Professional competency development arm of the curriculum addressing both the foundations of ethics and specific areas in ethics. The course includes basic ethical concepts and ethics in clinical settings.
	It aims at equipping the student with an overall understanding of medical ethics and law, the rights and duties of the medical profession and the rights of the patient and finally the legal provisions relating to the practice of medicine and of health professionals in general.
	Ethics will encourage the development of knowledge of duties of the graduate in promoting the health and medical welfare of the people they serve in ways which fairly and justly respect their dignity, autonomy and rights. These ethical issues are incorporated in all the curriculum years of the medical student.
Course Objectives	By the end of this unit, participants will be able to: 1. Describe the general scope of the field of medical ethics, including basic ethical principles 2. Explain the importance and utility of medical ethics 3. Describe the methodology of ethical deliberation 4. Analyse practical issues in the clinical setting from an ethics perspective 5. Describe some of the current areas of tension in bioethics
Course Content	1. Introduction: Definition of ethics; professional codes of ethics 2. Medical ethics: a) Historical overview b) Ethical theories c) Basic principles of medical ethics 3. Applicable Basic Principles of Law a) Ethics and the law b) Overview of health law in context country c) Context country's law on medical ethics. d) International laws and convention (Geneva, Nuremberg and Helsinki) 4. The Patient: A Person with Human and Other Legal Rights a) The doctor-patient relationship b) Communication c) Life and death

	d) End of life decisions: when, if ever, is it right to withhold treatment
	e) Breaking bad news and end of life care
	5. The Ethics of health policy
	a) Evidence for health policy
	b) The relationship between evidence and political values
	c) Equity and health maximization
	d) Accountability mechanisms
	6. Basic issues of medical ethics
	a) Codes of conduct
	b) Malpractice and negligence
	c) Confidentiality
	d) Irrational drug use
	e) Ethics of trust and right
	f) The issues related to the beginning and end of life
	g) Emerging issues including research and human experimentation
	h) Organ transplantation
	i) Genetics and AIDS
	7. Major Principles/Guidelines of Medical Ethics;
	a) Respect for patient autonomy
	b) Beneficence and justice
	c) Various perspectives to the application of medical ethics
	d) Considerations in the application of western medical ethics in developing countries
	e) Skepticism regarding medical ethics
	f) General code of ethics for context country's physicians
	g) Context country's medical association
	h) General code of ethics
	i) Six protocols for communicating bad news
Training Exercises	You are expected to put emphasis on demonstrations and role plays.
	• Role plays with examples and non-examples
	• Ethical dilemmas discussions
	• Small group discussions and debates
	• Case study discussions
	• Lectures
	• Demonstrations
	• Skill labs practice on standardized patients
	• Community and clinical situational analyses
	• Problem based learning
	• Self-directed learning (SDL)
	• E-Learning

Measurement based on Module Objectives	You may use any or all of the following:
	• DOCS (Direct Observation of Clinical Skills)
	• OSC/PE (Objective Structured Clinical / Practical Examination)
	• Oral exam (Viva)
	• Written exam (MCQ, Short Essay, Matching, True- False with reasoning) and portfolios
	• Project work
	• Quizzes and written tests
	• Assignments
	• Class / group presentations/ debates
	• Case presentations
	• Log books / Journals: Encourage the student to keep a weekly or monthly journal or course-based journal to enable him/her correlate all concepts which build into medicine.
	• Portfolios: Encourage the student to store all experiences (both successes and failures and make a continuous reflection on the topic).
	• **Summative assessment**
	  o Progressive (continuous) assessment (Quizzes, Concept application exercise tutorial-based evaluation) 40%
	  o End of each system exam 60%
	• **Formative assessment**
	  o This will not contribute to the total grade of the student but provides continuous feed back to the student and it can be applied in the form of providing feed backs on assignments completed and student's professional behaviour

Relevance to Course to other modules or Practice	• Good medical practice depends on mutual understanding and relationship between the doctor, the patient and the family with respect for patient's welfare, cultural diversity, beliefs and autonomy • Apply the principles of moral reasoning and decision-making to conflicts within and between ethical, legal and professional issues including those raised by economic constraints, commercialization of health care, and scientific advances; • Demonstrate self-regulation and recognition of the need for continuous self-improvement with an awareness of personal limitations including limitations of one's medical knowledge.

Student Hand-outs	• Provide hand-outs based on lecture notes, Trainer's research, audio-visual materials • Provide hand-outs compiled from collaborative and group work presentations • Individual research reports and case presentations may also be compiled for class references. • Give exercises to enable self-directed learning and compile the materials
Human Resources Required	• Clinicians • General Practitioner • Standardised patients • Other relevant Health Professionals (for Inter professional Pool)
Audio-Visual Materials / Special Equipment / Resources Required	• Small Group session smaller rooms. • Skills lab • Flip Charts • IT centre with good internet connection • Clinical set up • Library Multimedia equipment including: computer, LCD projector, Video, VCDs, DVDs, CD- ROMs • White board with white board marker or available resource • Electric power • Classroom or Lab
Reference Materials	1. Lo, Bernard. Resolving Ethical Dilemmas: *A Guide for Clinicians Fourth Edition, Lippincott,* Williams and Wilkins, 2009 2. Alora, Angeles, T. and Lumitao, (Eds.) (2001). *Beyond a Western Bioethics: Voices from the Developing World,* Georgetown University Press. 3. American College of Physicians. 1999. *Should doctors treat their relatives? (http://www.acponline.org/journals/news/jan99/relative.htm)* 4. American Medical Association. (2004). *Principles of medical ethics. (http://www.ama-assn.org/ama/pub/category/2512.html)* 5. Context country's Medical Association. (..............). *Medical Ethics for physicians Practicing in Context country.* 6. Joint United Nations Program on HIV/AIDS (UNAIDS) and World Health Organization (WHO). (1998). *Guidance Modules on Antiretroviral Treatments: Module 9. Ethical and Societal Issues Relating to Antiretroviral Treatments.* 7. Joint United Nations Program on HIV/AIDS (UNAIDS) and World Health Organization (WHO). (2004). *Guidance on Ethics and Equitable Access to HIV Treatment and Care.*

Professionalism

Course / Subject: Professionalism	
Course / Subject Time Distribution: Lectures - 2 Hours WGS - 2 Hours	
Course Objectives	On completion of this course student should be able to: 1. Identify values constructs foundational to the practice of medicine and the delivery of health care, including issues related to vulnerable and marginalized populations, and the recognition of cultural diversity using a broad definition and understanding of culture. 2. Demonstrate understanding of the importance of personal and professional ethics. 3. Describe laws, legislations and professional codes relevant to medical practice 4. Describe organizational structures applied within institutions and agencies accountable for the delivery of health care 5. Understand team versus hierarchical structures and understanding strategies for successful team functioning. 6. Have skills in negotiation and conflict resolution (*Adopted from McMaster University Health Sciences*)
Course Content	1. Values and constructs foundational to the practice of medicine 2. The delivery of health care, issues related to vulnerable and marginalized populations 3. Cultural diversity with a broad definition and understanding of culture 4. Personal and professional ethics, laws, legislations and professional codes relevant to medical practice 5. Organizational structures applied within institutions and agencies accountable for the delivery of health care 6. Team versus hierarchical structures and strategies for successful team functioning, negotiation and conflict resolution.
Training Exercises	You may use any of the following teaching and learning methods: • Team teaching with other experts • Project Research • Field trips • Community research • Lectures • Self-directed learning (SDL) • E-Learning • Demonstrations • Role plays

Measurement based on Module Objectives	You may use any or all of the following: • Unit Review Exercises • Project work / Assignments • Quizzes and written tests • Whole group / small group presentations • Journals: Encourage the student to keep a weekly or monthly journal or course-based journal to enable him/her correlate all concepts which build into medicine. • Portfolios: Encourage the student to store all experiences (both successes and failures and make a continuous reflection on the topic). • Summative assessments will be done at the end of the topic or module or semester.
Relevance to Course to other modules or Practice	This course will enable the student to demonstrate appropriate behaviours, habits and skills required for referral and consultation. It will also help the student to understand standards of care, institutional policies and standard operating procedures.
Student Hand-outs	• Provide a student's guide • Provide hand-outs based on lecture notes, Trainer's research, audio-visual materials • Provide hand-outs compiled from collaborative and group work presentations • Individual research and case presentation reports may also be compiled for class references. • Give exercises and hand-outs to enable self-directed learning
Audio-Visual Materials / Special Equipment / Resources Required	• Multimedia equipment including: computer, LCD projector, Video, VCDs, DVDs, CD- ROMs • White board with white board marker or available resource • Paper and hand-outs • Classroom or Lab
Reference Materials	Provide the student with Bibliographies, Websites, Library and E resources and relevant references.

Communication Skills

Course / Subject: Introduction to Communication Skills	
Course / Subject Time Distribution: Lectures - 3 Hours SGS - 3 Hours	
Course Description/ Design	The PCD component of the medical school curriculum intends to create student who not only have clinical skills but communication, ethics and professionalism. Communication is a basic clinical skill for all practice. The course will cover the most vital important communication skills for an effective patient-clinician interaction and quality health care: • Effective communication skills training can lead to improvement in patient and physician satisfaction and that it can significantly improve health care outcomes • The use of specific core skills make a difference in doctor-patient communication and its outcomes • An experiential skills-based training approach is an effective method to transform knowledge and attitudes into competent professional behaviour • Specific teaching methods are particularly effective in learning this skill, including observation, feedback, and reiteration.
Course Objectives	On completion of this course student should be able to: 1. Build and sustain a trusting relationship 2. Open the discussion 3. Gather information 4. Understand the patient's perspective 5. Share information 6. Reach agreement 7. Provide closure **The graduate will be competent in:** • Illustrating and linking concepts, principles and research evidence that support the importance and efficacy of developing communication and interpersonal skills in medicine. • Communication tasks and skills required to build a therapeutic relationship and to conduct an effective interview with the patient. • Communication tasks and skills required to communicate effectively about the patient. • Communication tasks and skills required to communicate effectively about medicine and science.

Course Content	1. Communication tasks in medicine and skills
	2. Channels of communication, communication barriers
	3. Effective communication
	4. Building and sustaining a trusting and professional relationship
	5. Open the discussion
	6. Gather information
	7. Understand the patient's perspective
	8. Share information
	9. Reach agreement
	10. Provide closure
Training Exercises	You may use any of the following teaching and learning methods during the communication skills training: • Role plays with non-examples, you are expected to put emphasis on demonstrations and role plays • Lectures • Demonstrations • Skill labs practice on standardized patients • Self-directed learning (SDL) • E-Learning • Hands on Training (HOT)
Measurement based on Module Objectives	You may use any or all of the following: • Skill demonstration • Practical exercises • Unit review exercises • Quizzes and written tests • Assignments • Class / group presentations • OSPEs and OSCEs • Summative assessments will be done at the end of the topic or module or semester.
Relevance to Course to other modules or Practice	This course will enable the medical student to gain competencies to effectively: • Interact with other professionals involved in patient care through effective teamwork • Demonstrate basic skills and positive attitudes towards teaching others • Demonstrate sensitivity to cultural and personal factors that improve interactions with patients and the community • Demonstrate appropriate behaviours, habits and skills required for referral and consultation • Understand standards of care, institutional policies and standard operating procedures

Student Hand-outs	• Provide a student's guide to enable the student to practice on their own. • Give exercises to enable self-directed learning
Audio-Visual Materials / Special Equipment / Resources Required	• Skills laboratory with standardized patients • Video recordings on effective communication • Multimedia equipment including: computer, LCD projector, Video, VCDs, DVDs, CD- ROMs • White board with white board marker or available resource • Paper and hand-outs
Reference Materials	Provide the student with Bibliographies, Websites, Library and E resources and relevant references.

Essentials of ICT Skills

Course / Subject: Essentials of ICT Skills	
Course / Subject Time Distribution: CRL - 8 Hours	
Course Design/ Description	This course covers basics concepts and skills training in Information Technology (IT) through to more advanced skills like using Windows, working with files and applications, and how to operate email and the internet.
	To prepare the student for e-learning, self-directed learning and use of IT for the learning process, the course presents the use and applications of ICT, hardware and software components of a computer, and how it is used for handling various types of documents, spread sheet, database, presentation, and how it's implemented for communicating and surfing the Internet.
	In Years 2-4 special IT skills will relate to specific areas SPH such as SPSS, STATA etc, Clinical and PCD such as health records EMR related will be offered. This course also provides clear connections on how all these functions are mapped to the health sector.
Course Objectives	On completion of this course student should be able to: 1. Describe and use basic ICT concepts 2. Show motivation for self-study 3. Identify and use computer hardware and software 4. Demonstrate and use basic application software such as MS-Word, MS-Excel, MS-Access, MS-PowerPoint, and Internet Explorer, and additional health related applications 5. Use Internet services 6. Keep confidentiality and security of health related electronic data 7. Respect ethical usage of internet service 8. Use health related software applications
Course Content	**Year 1: ICT** 1. Introduction to ICT 2. Windows operating system 3. Word processing 4. Spread sheet 5. Introduction to database 6. PowerPoint 7. Internet 8. Outlook **Year 2-4** 1. EMR 2. Biostatistics IT skills 3. SPSS, STATA

Training Exercises	You may use any of the following teaching and learning methods during the essentials of ICT Skills Training • Computer lab hands on • Lectures • Demonstration • Self-directed learning (SDL) • E-Learning • Hands on Training (HOT)
Measurement based on Module Objectives	You may use any or all of the following: • Take away quiz • Reading Assignments • Practical Exercises • Unit Review Exercises • Project work • Quizzes and written tests • Assignments • Class / group presentations • Journals: Encourage the student to keep a weekly or monthly journal or course-based journal to enable him/her correlate all concepts which build into medicine. • Portfolios: Encourage the student to store all experiences (both successes and failures and make a continuous reflection on the topic). • Summative assessments will be done at the end of the topic or module or semester.
Relevance to Course to other modules or Practice	This course will enable the graduate to: • Demonstrate effective ICT skills which will lead to improvement in accessing and researching significant universal practices of medicine. • ICT effective channel to transform knowledge and attitudes into competent professional behaviour.
Student Hand-outs	• Provide a student's guide to enable the student to practice on his/her own. • Give exercises to enable self-directed learning
Audio-Visual Materials / Special Equipment / Resources Required	• Fully equipped computer resource centre • Multimedia equipment including: computer, LCD projector, Video, VCDs, DVDs, CD- ROMs • White board with white board marker or available resource • Classroom or Lab • Paper and Hand-outs

Reference Materials	<ul><li>ECDL/ICDL Training Materials</li><li>Microsoft Office Manuals, Microsoft Corp, 2007</li><li>Office 2007 Bible by John Walkenbach, Wiley Publishing Inc, 2007</li><li>Introduction to Microsoft Windows XP by Liz Mortimer, University of Bradford, 2008</li><li>Concepts of Information Technology ECDL Module 1(Using XP) 1995-2004, Cheltenham Courseware Pty. Ltd</li><li>Microsoft Office 2007 Help Manual, http://www.brainbell. com.tutorials</li></ul>

Evidence Based Medicine

Course / Subject: Evidence Based Medicine	
Course / Subject Time Distribution: Lectures - 2 Hours WGS or CRL - 2 Hours	
Course Design/ Description	This course deals with evidence-based medicine (EBM) or evidence-based practice (EBP). It aims to orient the medical student to apply the best available evidence gained from scientific medicine to clinical decision making. It seeks to assess the strength of evidence of the risks and benefits of treatments (including lack of treatment) and diagnostic tests. Knowledge of EBM is important for the student to use EBM practice to provide care for his/her patients.
Course Objectives	By the end of this course the medical student should be able to: 1. Utilize principles of EBM in making decisions to provide treatment and care to his patients 2. Describe what EBM is and principles underlying it 3. Describe difference between guidelines and individual judgment in EBM 4. Describe the different levels of Evidences 5. Demonstrate use of EBM to improve patient care.

Course Content	1. Evolution of medical practice
	 2. Origins of medicine
	 3. Changes in practice based on different things ; change by thought leaders, feedback of outcomes
	 4. Systematic review of literature
	   a) At forefront: cardiology
	 5. Challenge of medicine:
	   a) Understanding of disease evolving
	   b) Expectation by society, patients, government, and colleagues that are informed.
	 6. Many practitioners were never trained in ebm; instead were taught from textbooks. Textbook issues:
	   a) Publishing lag time
	   b) Dependent on date of issue
	 7. What is the approach?
	   a) Not all patients are the same:
	     • 1st define question for inquiry
	     • Incidence or epidemiology
	     • Pathological or physiology
	     • Current diagnostic standards
	     • Management
	     • Complications
	     • Prognosis
	   b) Categorize inquiry as either foreground or background
	     • Background: Designed to improve general knowledge about a subject

| | o Examples:
   o What is the pathophysiology of lupus
   o What are the different types of lupus nephritis
• Good resources: textbooks, review articles
• Foreground: Patient-specific questions, strong implications for decisions, often with comparisons
  o Examples:
   o Which is the most sensitive test for lupus
   o For rapidly deteriorating lupus nephritis, which is the more effective medication-mycophenolate mofetil or cyclophosphamide
 c) Types of studies and guidelines:
  o Meta-analyses
  o Randomized control trials
  o Peer-reviewed journals
  o International Societies
8. Good Resources
 o Research databases
 o WHO Library, OVID, Pubmed, Cochrane Review, Google scholar, Faculty of 1000
9. Rating the evidence
 • Types of studies
  o Meta analysis
  o RCTs
  o Cohort Study
  o Case Control
  o Case Study
 • Analysis tools
 • Cross sectional vs. Longitudinal
 • Prospective vs. retrospective
 • Different types of bias
 • Selecting appropriate resources
10. Practicality:
 • Longitudinal cases
 • Presentation of paper |
| **Training Exercises** | You may use any of the following teaching and learning methods:
• Interactive lecture:
• Level of evidence
• Evidence-based guidelines
• Evidence-based individual decision making
• Exercise on identify level of evidence from lists of studies provided
• SGD, WGD
• Case study |

	• Case scenarios and suggested management plan versus evidence to support them • Case scenario and EBM and ethics of experimental or risky treatments • The rest of the content can be learnt by the student through individual study.
Measurement based on Module Objectives	• The student needs to have technology literacy to access to internet resources / shifts • You may grade groups with assurance of all group member participation • The student is required to conduct mini research projects and present findings in the format they have learnt (presentation of paper)
Relevance to Course to other modules or Practice	Through this course, the student will be competent in understanding and communicating the challenges of medicine; disease evolution / patterns; search, contribute and use credible evidence, practice within EBM and work within government and international practice guidelines.
Student Hand-outs	• Provide a student's guide to enable the student to practice on their own. • Provide hand-out detailing the lecture • Give exercises to enable student to gain research skills and paper presentation
Audio-Visual Materials / Special Equipment / Resources Required	• Computer resource centre with internet access • Video recordings on EBM presentations • Multimedia equipment including: computer, LCD projector, Video, VCDs, DVDs, CD- ROMs • White board with white board marker or available resource • Paper and hand-outs
Reference Materials	1. Guyatt, Gordon and Rennie, Drummond. *Users' Guide to the Medical Literature: Essentials of Evidence Based Clinical Practice American Medical Association* 2002 2. Jekel, Katz, Elmore. *Epidemiology, Biostatistics and Preventive Medicine,* Second Edition, W. B.Saunders, 2001 3. Sackett, Straus, Richardson, Rosenbert and Haynes. *Evidence Based Medicine* Second Edition, Churchill Livingstone, 2000

First Aid

Course / Subject: First Aid	
Course / Subject Time Distribution: WGS - 3 Hours	
Course Design/ Description	This course deals with training on problem solving in emergency situations. The student will gain knowledge on the limits of basic First Aid, Familiarize themselves with First Aid regulations and gain awareness of the duties of the employer / employee on issues of First Aid.
Course Objectives	By the end of this course, the medical student should be able to: 1. Demonstrate knowledge, skills and attitude in First Aid. Provide First Aid treatment in case of sudden illness or accidents using facilities or materials available to manage medical emergencies arising during practice and/or the environment.
Course Content	1. Principles of First Aid 2. Scope of First Aid 3. Assessing the situation 4. Making a diagnosis 5. Asphyxia and emergency resuscitation 6. Wounds and bleeding 7. Shock and fainting 8. Fractures 9. Use of splints and bandages 10. Burns and scalds 11. Poisoning and unconsciousness 12. Injuries to ligaments and joints 13. Safety at the workplace and highlights of accident prevention 14. Handling and transport of injured persons 15. Legal perspective of First Aid
Training Exercises	• Practical and theoretical examples • PowerPoint presentation • Video/DVD clips • SGD, WGD • Case studies • Case scenarios and suggested management plan versus evidence to support them • Case scenario and EBM and ethics of experimental or risky treatments • Class exercises • Handouts

Measurement based on Module Objectives	• Practical and theoretical tuition by First Aid instructor in basic first aid at the work place • Evaluation test leading to a Certificate in Basic First Aid, valid internationally for three years • Journals: Encourage the student to keep a weekly or monthly journal or course-based journal to enable him/her correlate all concepts which build into medicine • Portfolios: Encourage the student to store all experiences (both successes and failures and make a continuous reflection on the topic)
Relevance to Course to other modules or Practice	Through this course, the student will be competent in understanding and communicating the challenges of medicine; • Disease evolution / patterns • Search, contribute and use credible evidence • Practice within EBM and work within government and • International practice guidelines
Student Hand-outs	• Provide a learner's guide to enable the learner to practice on their own. • Provide handout detailing the lecture • Give exercises to enable student to gain research skills and paper presentation
Audio-Visual Materials / Special Equipment / Resources Required	• First Aid kits • Simulators • Manikins • Video recordings • Multimedia equipment including: computer, LCD projector, • Video, VCDs, DVDs, CD- ROMs • White board with white board marker or available resource • Paper and hand-outs
Reference Materials	1. Forgey, M. D. (2012). *Wilderness medicine: beyond first aid.* Rowman & Littlefield. 2. Van Tilburg, C. (Ed.). (2001). *First Aid: A Pocket Guide.* The Mountaineers Books. 3. Van Tilburg, C. (2001). *Emergency survival: a pocket guide: quick information for outdoor safety.* The Mountaineers Books.

Section IIB

Professional Competency Development

Clinical Skills Lab and Hospital OPD Practice

Duration: 40 Weeks (Years 1-4)

Demonstrations

You may use the following steps to prepare for demonstration lessons or laboratory sessions.

1. Develop demonstrations and role plays by breaking down the task into sequential steps (Task Analysis). You are expected do this for all procedures.
2. Once the steps are outlined, you **must** demonstrate the steps to the student either in the lab or in the clinic while the student observes.
3. Let the student practice the steps on his/her own
4. Ask the student to demonstrate the procedure for you / class
5. Give feedback at the end for correctly done procedures and any inconsistencies or missing links
6. Ask the student to practice again with the corrections
7. Each and every student **must** practice the skill.

Example I
Procedure/Task: Medical History Taking

There are two halves to each interview in medical history taking: **patient-centered** and **physician-centered**.

Physician-Centred
Physician's Agenda
Biomedical Focus
Physician Gathers Data

Patient-Centred
Patient's Agenda
Symptom Focus
Patient Tells Story

You may use the following outline for the interview:

1. The opening
2. Chief complaint(s) (CC)
3. History of present illness (HPI)
4. Primary
5. Secondary (focused review of systems ; ROS)
6. Tertiary (focused PMH)
7. Review of systems (ROS)
8. Past medical history (PMH)

Opening the Interview

It is important to begin each medical interview with a patient-centered approach.

1. Set the Stage
   - Welcome the patient - ensure comfort and privacy
   - Know and use the patient's name - introduce and identify yourself
2. Set the agenda
   - Use open-ended questions initially
   - Negotiate a list of **ALL** issues - avoid details
     - Chief complaint(s) and other concerns
     - Specific requests (i.e. medication refills)
   - Clarify the patient's expectations for this visit - ask the patient "Why now?"
3. Elicit the patient's story
   - Return to open-ended questions directed at the major problem (s)
   - Encourage with silence, nonverbal cues, and verbal cues
   - Focus by paraphrasing and summarizing
4. Make the Transition
   - Summarize the interview up to that point
   - Verbalize your intention to make a transition to the physician-centred interview

Primary History

Always start with the standard questions applied to the chief complaint (s):

1. Location
2. Radiation
3. Quality
4. Quantity
5. Duration
6. Frequency
7. Aggravating Factors
8. Relieving Factors
9. Associated Symptoms
10. Effect on Function

- Repeat this series of questions for each chief complaint. Ask one question at a time; avoid multi-part questions.
- Some questions won't work in certain situations, for example fatigue doesn't have a location.
- Record the information as objectively as possible without interpretation. Avoid medical jargon unless the patient uses it.
- Quote the patient directly as needed, "my teeth itch," for example.
- Pay close attention to the time course of the symptoms. Has symptom complex changed over time? This is particularly important with neurology, chest, and abdominal diseases.

Secondary History

The secondary history expands on the primary history, especially any associated symptoms. It is useful to think of the secondary history as a focused review of systems. These questions often bring out information that supports a certain diagnosis or helps gauge the severity of the disorder. Unlike the primary history, a certain amount of interpretation (and experience) is necessary. The following list should serve as a guide to get you started. It is incomplete and open to ideas and additions from you.

Fatigue
- Have the patient clarify exactly what they are experiencing.
- Ask about sleep. What is their "normal" pattern? Has this changed?

Fever
- Have they actually measured their temperature or just felt "hot?"
- Ask about chills or sweating.

Headache
- Be sure you understand the time course of the symptoms.
- Ask about nausea and vomiting.
- Ask about visual changes.
- Ask about the relationship with stress, work, week-ends, and emotions.

Eye Problems
- Ask about visual changes, loss of vision, blurring, or double vision
- Ask about spots, "floaters," or flashing lights.

Ear Problems
- Ask about hearing loss or ringing in the ears.
- Ask about dizziness or vertigo.
- For hearing loss, ask if they are having trouble understanding speech.
- Ask if anything has come out of the ear.

Nose Problems
- Is there is a seasonal pattern to the symptoms?
- Ask about any associated itching, especially of the eyes.

Chest Pain
- Ask about palpitations (awareness of heart beating), rapid pulse, or skipped beats.
- Has there been any shortness of breath? Is there any change when the patient lies down or sleeps? Does the patient sleep propped up on pillows or semi-upright in a chair?
- Ask if there is a relationship to activity. Has there been a change in exercise tolerance?
- Ask about swelling of the legs.

Cough
- Is the cough productive of sputum? What amount? What colour is it?
- Has there been any blood?

Abdominal Pain
- Be sure you understand the time course of the symptoms.
- Ask about nausea, vomiting, or loss of appetite.
- Ask about urinary symptoms. Has the urine changed colour?
- Ask about bowel habits. Have they changed? Is the stool black?

Joint Pain
- Is there any associated redness, swelling, heat, or loss of function?
- Ask about morning stiffness
- Ask about joint clicking or locking

Musculoskeletal Injury
- Ask precisely how the injury occurred
- Ask about loss of function, onset of swelling, and initial treatment

Tertiary History

The tertiary history brings in elements of the past medical history that have bearing on the patient's condition. By the time you get to the tertiary history you may already have a good idea of what might be going on. (This will be fine-tuned by the physical exam) Here are some examples:

Any HEENT or Chest Disorder
- Does the patient smoke? How much? How long?
- For children, does someone smoke in the home?

High Blood Pressure
- How much alcohol does the patient consume?

Breast Problems
- Is there a family history of breast cancer?

Depression
- Has the patient attempted suicide in the past?
- Has the patient been hospitalized in the past?

Abdominal Pain
- Does the patient smoke? How much? How long?
- How much alcohol does the patient consume?
- Prior to surgery, has the appendix been removed?

Chest Pain
- Does the patient smoke? How much? How long?
- Did the patient's parents die of a heart attack? At what ages?

Example II
Procedure/Task: Measuring Blood Pressure (Manually)

Using a sphygmomanometer and a stethoscope:

Introduce the equipment to the student.

- A sphygmomanometer is a device for measuring blood pressure. It includes an inflatable cuff, inflating bulb, and a gauge showing the blood pressure.
- The stethoscope has 2 earpieces, tubing, and a diaphragm (flat disk at the end). It is used for listening to sounds from the body. Carefully read the directions before using your blood pressure kit.
- Each blood pressure kit may have variations. However, the following steps may be helpful in training the student to take a blood pressure:

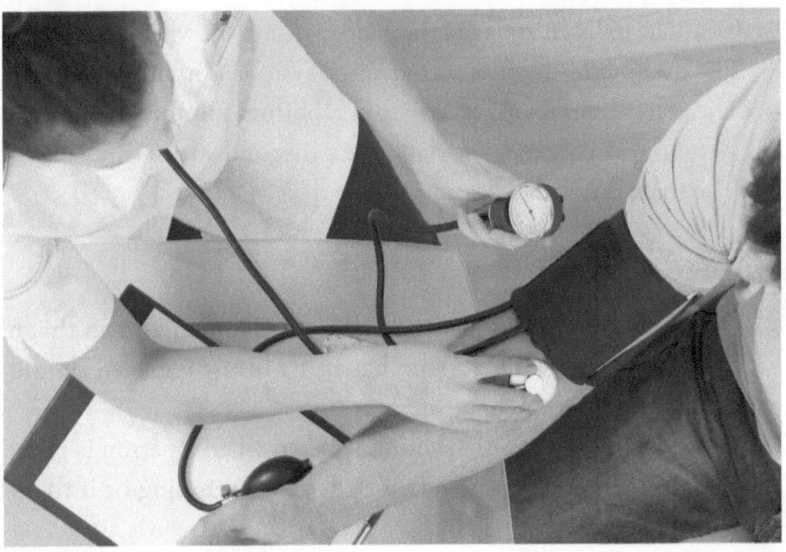

1. Prepare the patient.
2. Sit up or lie down with the arm stretched out. The arm should be level with the heart.
3. Put the cuff about 1 inch (2.5 cm) above the elbow. Wrap the cuff snugly around the arm. The blood pressure reading may not be correct if the cuff is too loose.
4. Put the earpieces in your ears.

Using your middle (long) and index (pointer) fingers, gently feel for the pulse in the bend of the elbow. This is the brachial artery. You will feel the pulse beating when you find it. Do not use your thumb to feel for the pulse because your thumb has a pulse of its own.

5. Put the diaphragm of the stethoscope over the brachial artery pulse. Listen for the heartbeat.
6. Tighten the screw on the bulb and quickly squeeze and pump the bulb. This will cause the cuff to tighten.
7. Keep squeezing the bulb until the scale on the gauge reads about 160. Or, until the gauge reads at least 10 points higher than when you last hear the heartbeat.
8. Slowly loosen the screw to let air escape from the cuff. Let the gauge fall about 5 points a second. Carefully look at the gauge and listen to the sounds. Remember the number on the gauge where you first heard the thumping sound.
9. Continue to listen and read the gauge at the point where the sound stops.
10. The number of the first sound is the systolic (top number) pressure.
11. The second number is the diastolic (bottom number) pressure.
12. Write down your BP, the date, the time, and which arm was used to take the BP. Let the air out of the cuff.

Helpful Tips:

1. Do not take a blood pressure on an injured arm or an arm that has an IV or a shunt. A woman who has had a breast removed should have her BP taken on the opposite arm
2. Usually a blood pressure should be taken when a person is rested and relaxed. It should not be taken right after exercising or if the person is feeling stressed
3. Ask the person to sit or lie down for about 2 minutes with the arm stretched out. The patient should be relaxed
4. If you are unable to feel the pulse, try using the stethoscope
5. Put the diaphragm of the stethoscope over the bend in the arm
6. Tighten the screw on the bulb. Squeeze the bulb of the cuff until you see the number 160 on the blood pressure gauge. Slowly loosen the screw on the bulb and listen for the pulse.

7. You may need to move the diaphragm around a bit until you find the pulse. If you cannot hear the pulse, check the reading of the last blood pressure.
8. Then, pump the cuff 10 to 20 points higher than that reading.

Additional teaching and learning methods

Role Plays

When you plan to use role plays:
1. Be clear on the objective of what is to be achieved
2. Break the concepts to see how they relate with each other
3. Write a script with a maximum of three characters
4. Act it out before taking it to the classroom
5. In the classroom, explain the objective to the student
6. Ask the student to act out
7. Discuss the play with the student to understand what they have learned.
8. Explain the objective again giving examples and non-examples.

Time Table for Professional Competency Development for CVS: Clinical Skills Lab and Hospital OPD Practice

Week	Objective/ Activity	Teaching/ Learning Methods	Learning Site/Time		Resource Needed
			Skill Lab	Hospital	
Wk 1	Take history from a patient suspected of cardiovascular disorder	Demonstration, role play, coaching, and observation in hospital	2 hrs	1 hr	Script for role play Learning guide and checklist for history taking
	Conduct physical examination of the CVS/ Stethoscope use and measuring BP	Demonstration, role play, coaching	1 hr	-	Learning guide and checklist for P/E Stethoscope and BP apparatus
Wk 2	Take history from a patient suspected of cardiovascular disorder	Observation, practice and coaching	-	1 hr	Learning guide and checklist for history taking
	Perform physical examination of the CVS/examination of the pericardium, pulse, and jugular venous pressure	Demonstration, video show, role play, coaching	3 hrs		DVD/VCD on P/E of the CVS Stethoscope Learning guide and checklist on P/E of the CVS Computer and LCD projector (or TV and DVD player) Ruler Examination coach
Wk 3	Take history from a patient suspected of cardiovascular disorder	Observation, practice and coaching		1 hr	Learning guide and checklist for history taking

	Objective	Method	Duration	Materials
	Perform and/or interpret basic diagnostic procedures (Recording and reading normal ECG; basic reading of chest X-ray in relation to the heart; Recognize normal heart on echocardiography)	Practice ECG recording and basic reading Demonstration and practice basic reading of chest X-ray Demonstration of Echo video or photographs	3 hrs	ECG machine ECG records of abnormal heart Sample chest X-ray films (normal and abnormal heart) Video and/or images of echocardiogram Examination coach
Wk 4	Practice and perform life-saving and surgical procedures in a simulated setting (Use of puls-oximetry; administering oxygen using different gadgets; use defibrillator; venous cut-down)	Demonstration, video show, practice on models	3 hrs –	Puls-oximetry Oxygen source, mask, nasal catheter and ambu bag Defibrillator (or video of defibrillator) DVD/VCD of defibrillation Computer and LCD projector (or TV and DVD player) Venous cut-down set
	Perform physical examination of the CVS	Observation in hospital OPD, practice and coaching	1 hr	Learning guide and checklist Stethoscope Ruler
Wk 5	Practice basic cardiopulmonary resuscitation	Video show, demonstration, practice on models, coaching	3 hrs	DVD/VCD of CPR Computer and LCD projector (or TV and DVD player) Oxygen source, mask, nasal catheter and ambu bag

Week	Objective	Method	Time	Resources
				Laryngoscope and endotracheal tube Mannequin Learning guide and checklist
	Perform physical examination of the CVS	Observation in hospital OPD, practice and coaching	1 hr	Learning guide and checklist Stethoscope, Ruler
Wk 6	Practice pericardiocentesis in a simulated setting	Video show, practice on models, coaching	1 hr	DVD/VCD of pericardiocentesis Computer and LCD projector (or TV and DVD player) Pericardiocentesis procedure model and set Learning guide and checklist
	Discuss ethical issues related to care of a patient to cardiovascular disorder	Case-based discussion	2 hrs.	Case studies
	Perform physical examination of the CVS	Observation in hospital OPD, practice and coaching	1 hr	Learning guide and checklist Stethoscope Ruler

N.B.

- The student should utilize all opportunities for observing and assisting life-saving and surgical procedures at the hospital throughout the module.
- Student must have achieved competency of the desired clinical skills in simulated setting before they can work on patients.

Social and Population Health (Guide)

Section III

Social Population Health and Health Systems

Duration: 24 Weeks

Course Description

Social and population health (SPH) is a composite of integrated modules, community placement and primary health care units attachment designed to equip the student with the required knowledge, skills and attitude to:

1. Apply principles and methods of public health to prevent disease and
2. Promote health of individuals, families and communities in collaboration with the community and other sectors.

Course Design

SPH is delivered longitudinally throughout the years of training and organized into four components. The first one is SPH modules will comprise of classroom and community learning experiences. The modules are organized thematically:

1. determinants of health (SPH-I)
2. measurement of health and disease (SPH-II)
3. health promotion and disease prevention (SPH-III)
4. health policy and management (SPH-IV) and
5. research methodology (SPH-V)

The second component is a community-based training program (CBTP), which occurs at the end of the pre-clerkship modules in year two. The third component is a team training program (TTP), which is a service-learning, where medical interns are deployed in primary health care units with other healthcare cadres for clinical as well as community health work.

The fourth component, student research project, will be part of the internship program.

Relevance to medical practice is given due emphasis all along.

Social and Population Health (Guide)

Section IIIA

Social Population Health and Health Systems

Social and Population Health –I

Determinants of Health

Determinants of Health

Course / Subject: SPH Determinants of Health	
Course / Subject Time Distribution: 24 weeks • Classroom: Every Thursday, 8-10 AM, for 24 weeks • PHCU/Community visit: Every Friday, 8:30-12:30 AM, for 24 weeks	
Course Design/ Description	This first SPH module is designed to equip the medical student with the knowledge, skills and attitude needed to analyse determinants of population health with full participation of the community. The SPH-I module is offered in parallel with integrated biomedical and professional competency development modules during the first pre-clerkship year. Classroom sessions are interwoven with community and PHCU-based experiences to reinforce understanding, apply new knowledge, and develop practical competencies.
Course Objectives	By the end of this module, the medical student will be able to: • Analyse broad determinants of health and disease at individual, family and community level in collaboration with them. **Learning Objectives** 1. Describe the notion of health and disease as a whole and by components (physical, mental, and social) at individual, family and community level 2. Describe the history, development, basic concepts, principles and sciences in public health 3. Analyse important social, cultural, economic, psychological, behavioural, environmental, and nutritional determinants of health and illness of communities 4. Communicate effectively with individuals, families, communities, PHCU staff, local health department staff, peers and faculty 5. Interact with individuals and families with sensitivity to personal and cultural factors 6. Advise individuals and families to prevent and control health risks and determinants 7. Demonstrate professional values and behaviour in interaction with individuals, families and communities consistent with the future role of a physician

	8. Demonstrate key public health values, attitudes and behaviours such as commitment to equity and social justice, recognition of the importance of the health of the community as well as the individual, and respect for diversity, self-determination, empowerment, and community participation
	9. Show respect for colleagues and other healthcare professionals and the ability to foster a positive collaborative relationship with them
	10. Analyse community practice experience and perform practice-based improvement activities using a systematic methodology.
	11. Use information technology to manage information, access online medical information, and support one's own education.
	12. Demonstrate a habit of self-reflection, responsiveness to feedback and an on-going development of new skills, knowledge and attitude.
	13. Search, collect, organize and interpret health and health-related information from different sources
	14. Able to use information and communication technology to assist in health promotion and disease prevention measures for individuals, and families.
Course Content	1. Introduction to public health • Health and disease: concepts, definitions and perspectives • Public health: definition, philosophy, history, development, core functions and services • Public health sciences, their scope and use in medicine • Organization of health services in Context country 2. Socio-economic determinants of health • Socio-cultural factors including, but not limited to, place of residence, urbanization, culture, religion, ethnicity, gender views and roles, status of women, educational status, demography, social structures (mobility and migration) and organizations (social cohesion, support and network), laws, human rights • Economic factors such as unemployment, poverty, income inequality, neighborhood deprivation, assets, economic growth, globalization, healthcare cost

	3. Psychosocial and behavioural determinants of health • Developmental psychology • Personality and health • Overview of relationship between health and human behaviour (sexual practices, smoking, alcohol, exercise) • Ecology and environmental determinants of health • Human and environment • Ecological model of health and disease • Biosphere and pollution • Environment and health • Housing and institutional sanitation • Water sanitation • Waste disposal • Vector control • Food sanitation • Occupational health and safety • Nutrition and health • Introduction to human nutrition • Mechanisms and principles underlying nutritional health, and malnutrition • Nutritional requirements at different stages of the life cycle • Common food sources of nutrients and nutritional anthropology in Context country • Assessment of dietary intake • Assessment of nutritional status • Epidemiology and consequences of malnutrition in Context country (child malnutrition and maternal malnutrition) • Macronutrient deficiencies of public health importance in Context country • Micronutrient deficiencies of public health importance in Context country • Public health interventions to address malnutrition • Food and nutrition policies and programs in Context country
Training Exercises	• Interactive lecture and discussion • Small group learning activities: assignment, exercise, case study • Individual reading

	• PHCU/Community-based learning and study trip: home visit, discussion with individuals and families to identify and solve problems, observation, PHCU visit, Zonal and District Health Department Visit, field visit, and targeted literature review based on community experience • Student presentation • Personal research and reflection exercise (PRRE) • Reflective portfolio and mentoring
Measurement based on Module Objectives	**Formative assessment** • Exercise and assignment • Logbook and portfolio • 360 degree evaluation • Student presentation • Global rating of community experience midway during the module **Summative assessment** • Written exam (50 %) • PRRE (15 %) • Reflective portfolio (10 %) • Global rating of community experience (15 %) • Assignment and student presentation (10 %)
Relevance to Course to other modules or Practice	This course will enable the graduate to: • Demonstrate key public health values, attitudes and behaviours such as commitment to equity and social justice, recognition of the importance of the health of the community as well as the individual, and respect for diversity, self-determination, empowerment, and community participation • Describe the principles, scope and uses of public health sciences and methods in medicine • Demonstrate cultural competency required to interact with diverse individuals and communities • Synthesize and present information appropriate to the needs of the audience, and discuss achievable and acceptable plans of action that address issues of priority to the individual and community • Exercise appropriate utilization of human resources, diagnostic interventions, therapeutic modalities and health care facilities

	• Analyse important life-style, genetic, demographic, environmental, social, economic, psychological, and cultural determinants of health and illness of a population as a whole • Describe global and national trends in morbidity and mortality of diseases of public health significance, the impact of migration, trade, and environmental factors on health and the role of international health organizations • Identify, formulate and solve community health problems using scientific thinking and based on obtained and correlated information from different sources
Student Hand-outs	• Provide a student's guide • Give exercises to enable self-directed learning • Hard or soft copy hand-outs
Audio-Visual Materials / Special Equipment / Resources Required	• LCD and computer or Overhead projector and transparencies, • White board and available resources • Handouts of lecture materials • Logbooks for entry of community experience
Reference Materials	As applicable to your context

Teaching-Learning Methods

- Interactive lecture
- Active learning activities
- Role plays
- Adapted puzzles and games
- Problem based learning (PBL)
- Scenario based learning
- Small group sessions
- Whole group session
- Skills lab and Integrated biomedical laboratory practical session
- Community learning sessions
- E-learning
- Mentorship
- Self-directed learning

Assessments

Summative Assessment
- Progressive (continuous) assessment (Quizzes, concept application exercises, tutorial-based evaluation) 40%
- End of each system exam 60%

Formative Assessment
- This will not contribute to the total grade of the student but provides continuous feed back to the student and it can be applied in the form of providing feed backs on assignments completed, student' professional behaviour.

Methods of Assessment
- OSPE (Objective Structured Practical Exam)
- PRRE (Personal Research and Reflection Exercise)
- Project Presentation
- Oral exam (Viva)
- Written exam (MCQ, Short Essay, Matching, True- False with reasoning)
- Log books and portfolios

Resources Needed

Human resources
- Biomedical specialist
- Clinicians
- General Practitioner
- Other relevant health professionals (for Inter professional pool)
- Education Experts

Training, leaching and learning materials
- Trainer's Guide
- Reference manuals and books
- Student Guide
- Handout

- Books
- Text books
- E-books
- Online and physical libraries

Learning Facilities / Infrastructure
- Class rooms
- Small group session smaller rooms.
- Skills lab
- Dissection room
- Equipped laboratories s for respective departments
- IT centre with good internet connection
- Clinical set up (primary and secondary where possible tertiary care health institutions)
- Library / Resource centre

Portable and stationary plants, machines and equipment
- Flip charts
- Video cassette
- CD-ROM
- Computers
- DVD Player
- LCD projector Overhead Projector
- White board (2x1.5)

www.ingramcontent.com/pod-product-compliance
Lightning Source LLC
Chambersburg PA
CBHW021959170526
45157CB00003B/1057